Health Policy Issues

An Economic Perspective on Health Reform

AUPHA Press
Health Administration Press

Editorial Board

Howard S. Zuckerman, Chair
Arizona State University

Farrokh Alemi
Cleveland State University

James M. Carman
University of California, Berkeley

Jan P. Clement
Virginia Commonwealth University

David J. Fine
Tulane University

Judith R. Lave
University of Pittsburgh

Joel M. Lee
University of Kentucky

Mary Richardson
University of Washington

Sam B. Sheps
University of British Columbia

AUPHA Press/Health Administration Press is a cooperative publishing activity of the Association of University Programs in Health Administration and the Foundation of the American College of Healthcare Executives.

Health Policy Issues

An Economic Perspective on Health Reform

Paul J. Feldstein

AUPHA Press/Health Administration Press
Ann Arbor, Michigan   1994

RA
410.53
F 455
1994

Copyright © 1994 by the Foundation of the American College of Healthcare Executives. Printed in the United States of America. All rights reserved. This book or parts thereof may not be reproduced in any form without written permission of the publisher. Opinions and views expressed in this book are those of the author and do not necessarily reflect those of the Foundation of the American College of Healthcare Executives or the Association of University Programs in Health Administration.

98   97   96   95   94   5   4   3   2   1

Library of Congress Cataloging-in-Publication Data

Feldstein, Paul J.
  Health policy issues : an economic perspective / Paul J. Feldstein.
     p.   cm.
  Includes bibliographical references and index.
  ISBN 1-56793-019-0
  1. Medical economics—United States.   2. Medical care—United States—Cost control.   3. Medical care, Cost of—United States.   4. Insurance, Health—United States.
I. Title.
RA410.53.F455   1994   338.4'33621'0973—dc20   94-20620 CIP

The paper used in this publication meets the minimum requirements of American National Standard for Information Sciences—Permanence of Paper for Printed Library Materials, ANSI Z39.48-1984. ∞™

Health Administration Press
A division of the Foundation
  of the American College of
  Healthcare Executives
1021 East Huron Street
Ann Arbor, Michigan 48104
(313) 764-1380

Association of University Programs
  in Health Administration
1911 North Fort Myer Drive, Suite 503
Arlington, VA 22209
(703) 524-5500

OCT 03 1994
Lamont Library
Harvard University

*To my friends and
colleagues at Sutter Health*

Table of Contents

List of Figures

List of Tables

Preface

I have often given lectures on the implications of the changing health care system to hospital boards of trustees, medical groups, and, more recently, to medical students. Afterward I am usually asked to provide references that would allow the interested listener to pursue a particular subject in greater depth. My response has been to suggest a few journals that are not technical and contain short articles. Many in my audience would like to learn more about particular subjects, but they have limited time to spend. I have always apologized for not being able to provide a simple reference that includes material on a variety of additional topics of interest to my listeners.

Being an economist, I believe that an economic approach is very useful, not only for understanding the forces pressuring for change in health care but also for explaining why the health system has evolved to its current state. Even the political issues surrounding the financing and delivery of health services can be better understood when viewed through an economic perspective, that is, the economic self-interest of participants.

It is for these reasons that I believe there is a need for an issue-oriented book, containing short discussions on each subject, and using an economic perspective. The economic perspective used throughout is that of a "market" economist, namely, one who believes that markets—in which suppliers compete for customers on the basis of price and quality— are the most effective mechanisms for allocating resources. Of course, at times markets fail, or lead to outcomes that are undesirable in terms of equity. Market economists generally believe that government economic interventions, no matter how well intentioned or carefully thought out, can neither replicate the efficiency with which markets allocate resources, nor fully anticipate the behavioral responses of the economic agents affected by the intervention. In cases of market failure, market economists prefer solutions that fix the underlying problem while retaining basic market incentives rather than replacing the market altogether with government planning or provision.

The current debate on health care reform is unlikely to be concluded once specific proposals are enacted. Any subject affecting the lives of so many and requiring such a large portion of our country's resources will continue to be a topic of debate and legislative change. Hopefully, this book will help to clarify some of the more significant issues.

To help the reader focus on important points related to each issue, a list of discussion questions for each chapter is included at the end of the book.

I thank Thomas Wickizer for his collegial support, Jerry German, and two anonymous reviewers for their comments, Nasir Kamal for data collection and construction of figures, and Greta Brooks for editorial assistance.

1

The Rise in Medical Expenditures

The rapid growth in medical expenditures over the past 25 years is as familiar as the increasing percent of our GNP devoted to medical care. Less well known are the reasons for this continual rise in medical expenditures. The purpose of this introductory chapter is twofold: to provide an historical perspective to the medical sector and to explain the rise in medical expenditures within an economic framework.

Before Medicare and Medicaid

Until 1965, spending in the medical sector was predominately private—80 percent of all expenditures were spent by individuals out-of-pocket or by private health insurance on their behalf. The remaining expenditures were paid by the federal government (8.4 percent) and the states (12 percent) (see Table 1.1). Total medical expenditures were $36 billion and represented approximately 6 percent of our gross national product (GNP), that is, 6 cents out of every dollar spent was for medical services.

Effects of Medicare and Medicaid

In 1965 two major government programs, Medicare and Medicaid, were enacted, which dramatically increased the role of government in the financing of medical care. Medicare covered the aged and consisted of two parts: Part A was for hospital care and was financed by a Social Security tax on the working population. Part B covered physicians' services

Table 1.1   Personal Health Care Expenditures by Source of Funds, 1965 and 1991

Source of Funds	1965 (in billions)	(%)	1991 (in billions)	(%)
Total	$35.6	100.0%	$660.2	100.0%
Private	28.4	79.6	377.0	57.1
Out-of-pocket	19.0	53.4	144.3	21.9
Insurance benefits	8.7	24.3	209.3	31.7
All other	0.7	1.9	23.4	3.5
Public	7.3	20.4	283.3	42.9
Federal	3.0	8.4	204.1	30.9
State and local	4.3	12.0	79.1	12.0

Sources: S. W. Letsch, H. C. Lazenby, K. R. Levit, and C. A. Cowan, "National Health Expenditures, 1991," *Health Care Financing Review* 14 (Winter 1992): 1–29; Office of National Cost Estimates, "National Health Expenditures, 1988," *Health Care Financing Review* 11 (Summer 1990): 1–41.

and was financed from both federal taxes (currently 75 percent) and by the aged themselves (25 percent). Medicaid was for the categorically or medically needy, which included indigent aged and families with dependent children receiving cash assistance. Each state administered its program, and the federal government paid, on average, more than half of the costs. As a result of Medicare and Medicaid, the federal government became a major payer of medical services.

In 1991, 43 percent of total medical expenditures were paid by the government, with the federal share being 31 percent and the states at 12 percent. The private share declined to 57 percent, with only 22 percent paid out-of-pocket. The rapid increase in total health expenditures is illustrated in Table 1.2, which shows expenditures on the different components of medical services over time. Figure 1.1 shows where the health care dollar comes from and how it is distributed among the different health care providers.

The United States spent over $900 billion, more than 14 percent of our GNP, on medical care in 1993, and these expenditures are rising at 11–12 percent per year (Letsch 1993). If this rate continues, then medical spending will reach $1.6 trillion and comprise more than 18 percent of GNP by the year 2000.

Table 1.2   National Health Expenditures, Selected Calendar Years,
1965–1991 (billions of dollars)

	1965	*1970*	*1980*	*1990*	*1991*
Total national health expenditures	$41.6	$74.4	$250.1	$675.0	$751.8
Health services and supplies	38.2	69.1	238.9	652.4	728.6
Personal health care	35.6	64.9	219.4	591.5	660.2
Hospital care	14.0	27.9	102.4	258.1	288.6
Physician services	8.2	13.6	41.9	128.8	142.0
Dental services	2.8	4.7	14.4	34.1	37.1
Other professional services	0.9	1.5	8.7	30.7	35.8
Home health care	0.1	0.1	1.3	7.6	9.8
Drugs, medical nondurables	5.9	8.8	21.6	55.6	60.7
Vision products, other medical durables	1.2	2.0	4.6	11.7	12.4
Nursing home care	1.7	4.9	20.0	53.3	59.9
Other personal health care	0.8	1.4	4.6	11.5	14.0
Program administration and net cost of private health insurance	1.9	2.8	12.2	38.9	43.9
Government public health activities	0.6	1.4	7.2	22.0	24.5
Research and construction	3.5	5.3	11.3	22.7	23.1
Research	1.5	2.0	5.4	11.9	12.6
Construction	1.9	3.4	5.8	10.8	10.6
National health expenditures per capita	$204	$346	$1,064	$2,601	$2,868

Sources: S. W. Letsch, H. C. Lazenby, K. R. Levit, and C. A. Cowan, "National
Health Expenditures, 1991," *Health Care Financing Review* 14 (Winter 1992): 1–29;
H. C. Lazenby and S. W. Letsch, "National Health Expenditures, 1989," *Health Care
Financing Review* 12 (Summer 1990): 1–26.

Medical expenditures consist of prices multiplied by quantity of
services. The rise in medical expenditures can be explained by looking
at the factors that lead to changes in medical prices and quantities. In a
market system, prices and output of goods and services are determined by
the interaction of buyers (the demand side) and sellers (the supply side)
in a market. We can analyze changes in prices and output by examining
how various interventions change the behavior of buyers and sellers. One
such intervention was Medicare, which lowered the out-of-pocket price
the aged had to pay for medical care. The result was a dramatic increase

Figure 1.1   The Nation's Health Care Dollar, 1991

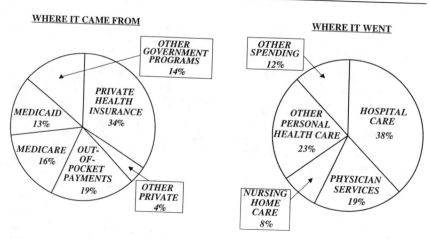

"Other personal health care" includes dental care, vision care, home health care, drugs, medical products, and other professional services.

"Other spending" includes program administration, net cost of private health insurance, government public health, research, and construction.

Source: S. W. Letsch, H. C. Lazenby, K. R. Levit, and C. A. Cowan, "National Health Expenditures, 1991," *Health Care Financing Review* 14 (Winter 1992): 1–29.

in the demand for hospital and physician services by the aged, leading to a dramatic increase in prices and, to a lesser amount, an increase in use of those services. Total expenditures increased since the higher prices multiplied by the greater quantity equaled a higher level of expenditures.

When costs, which underlie the supply of any service, increase, prices also increase. As hospitals tried to attract more nurses to care for the increased demands by the aged, they had to raise nurses' wages, which were then passed on in higher hospital prices. Similarly, government payments for the poor under Medicaid increased their demands for medical services. The result of increased demands for care and higher costs of providing that care was rapidly rising expenditures.

At the same time that the government was subsidizing the demands of the aged and poor, the demand for medical services by the employed population was increasing. Stimulating the growth in private health insurance during the late 1960s and 1970s was the growth in incomes, the high marginal income tax rates (up to 70 percent), and the high inflation rate in the economy. The high inflation rate was pushing more people into higher marginal tax brackets. Receiving additional income in the form of wages, and then paying federal, state, and Social Security taxes, would leave the employee with less disposable income to spend, up to 50 percent less if they were in a 50 percent marginal income tax bracket. Instead of having the employer pay wage increases in after-tax cash, which could be taxed at 50 percent, the employee chose to have the employer spend those same dollars, before tax, to buy additional health insurance. Thus the employee could have their out-of-pocket medical expenses paid with before-tax dollars rather than after-tax dollars. This tax subsidy for employer-paid health insurance stimulated the demand for medical services in the private sector and further increased medical prices.

Demand increased most rapidly for those medical services that were covered by government and private health insurance. Currently only 5.5 percent of hospital care and 19 percent of physician services is paid out-of-pocket by the patient; the remainder is paid for by some third party. Patients had little incentive to be concerned with the price of the service when they were not responsible for paying a significant portion of the price. As the out-of-pocket price declined, the use of services increased.

The aged, who represent 12 percent of the population and use more medical services than any other age group, filled 40 percent of hospital beds. And use of physician services by the aged, the poor, and those with insurance also increased.

Advances in medical technology led to a further stimulus in demands for medical treatment. New methods of diagnosis and treatment were developed; those with previously untreatable diseases could now have access to technology that offered hope of a recovery from illness. And new diseases, such as AIDS, led to further demands on the medical system. These dramatic increases in third party payments (both public and private), an aging population, and new technologies led to increases in both prices and quantities of medical services.

Providers (hospitals and physicians) responded to these increased demands for care. However, the method by which they responded unnecessarily increased the cost of providing medical services. When Medicare was enacted, hospitals were paid their costs plus 2 percent for serving Medicare patients. Hospitals, which were predominantly not-for-profit, consequently expanded their capacity, invested in the latest technology, and duplicated facilities and services available in nearby hospitals. There were few incentives for hospitals to be efficient since they were reimbursed their costs. Hospital prices rose faster than any other medical service. Similarly, physicians had little cause for concern over hospital costs. Physicians wanted their hospital to have the latest equipment so that they would not have to refer their patient elsewhere (and possibly lose them); they would hospitalize their patient for diagnostic workups and keep their patients longer in the hospital since it was less costly *for the patient* covered by hospital insurance. Outpatient services, which were less costly than hospital care, were generally not covered by third party payers.

In addition to the lack of patient incentives to be concerned with the cost of their care and the similar lack of provider incentives for supplying that care efficiently, restrictions were imposed by the government on the delivery of services. Under both Medicare and Medicaid the government was not permitted to contract with organizations, such as health maintenance organizations (HMOs), to deliver care on an annual capitation payment. Organized medicine was instrumental in having included in both Medicare and Medicaid the concept of "free choice of physician." Organizations, such as HMOs, that preclude their enrollees from choosing any physician in the community would violate the "free choice of physician" rule and were thus unable to receive capitation payments from the government. There were also numerous state restrictions on HMOs that further inhibited their development. These restrictions made it impossible for the government (and difficult for private insurers) to contract with closed panels of providers that were less expensive.

The effect of increased demands, limited patient and provider incentives to search for lower-cost approaches, together with restrictions on the delivery of medical services, resulted in rapidly rising prices, increased use of services, and, consequently, greater medical expenditures.

Government Response to Rising Costs

As expenditures under Medicare and Medicaid increased, the federal government faced limited options: (1) it could raise Social Security and income taxes on the non-aged to continue funding these programs, (2) it could require the aged to pay higher premiums for Medicare and increase their deductibles and copayments, or (3) the government could reduce their payments to hospitals and physicians. Each of these approaches would cost the government political support from some constituency, such as employees, the aged, or health care providers. The least politically costly options appeared to be to increase taxes on the non-aged and to pay hospitals and physicians less.

Additional regulatory approaches were also used by the federal and state governments to control these rapidly rising expenditures. Medicare utilization review programs were instituted, and controls were placed on hospital investment in new facilities and equipment. These government controls proved ineffective as hospital expenditures continued their rapid rise throughout the 1970s. The government then limited physician fee increases under Medicare and Medicaid, with the consequence that many physicians refused to participate in these programs. Access to care by the poor decreased. And as physicians refused to participate in Medicare, many Medicare patients had to pay higher out-of-pocket fees if they were to be seen by physicians.

In 1979 President Carter's highest domestic priority was to enact expenditure limits on Medicare hospital cost increases; he was defeated by a Congress controlled by his own political party.

The 1980s

By the beginning of the 1980s, there was no political consensus on what should be done to control increases in Medicare hospital and physician expenditures. And private health expenditures were also continuing their rapid rise. Yet by the mid-1980s strong cost-containment pressures were being imposed on both the Medicare and private medical sectors.

Several events occurred in the early 1980s that brought major changes to the medical sector. The HMO legislation, which was enacted in 1974, began to have its effect in the 1980s. In 1974 President Nixon wanted a health program that would not increase federal expenditures. The result was the HMO Act of 1974, which legitimized HMOs and removed restrictive state laws retarding the development of federally approved HMOs. Unfortunately, many HMOs decided not to seek federal qualification because there were restrictions that would have caused their premiums to be too high, and thereby not price competitive with traditional health insurers. These restrictions were removed by the late 1970s and the growth of HMOs began in the early 1980s.

To achieve savings in Medicaid, the Reagan administration in 1981 removed the "free choice of provider" requirement for Medicaid enrollees; states were able to require their Medicaid population to participate in closed provider panels. The states were then able to contract with HMOs and accept bids from hospitals for care of their Medicaid patients. (The "free choice" requirement remained in place for the aged until the mid-1980s, when the aged were permitted to voluntarily join HMOs.)

Federal subsidies to expand the number of medical school spaces, which were enacted in 1964, began to have their effect on the supply of physicians: the number of physicians expanded from 145 per 100,000 population in 1965 to 200 per 100,000 in 1980; it reached 240 per 100,000 in 1990. The increased supply of physicians made it easier for HMOs to attract physicians and to expand their capacity and also to dampen increases in physician fees.

A new Medicare hospital payment system was phased in during 1983. Hospitals were no longer to be paid according to their costs; fixed prices were established for each diagnostic admission (referred to as DRGs), and an annual limit was set on the increase in these fixed prices per admission each year. DRG prices changed hospitals' incentives. Since hospitals could keep the difference between their costs and the fixed DRG price, they now had an incentive to reduce their costs for caring for Medicare patients and to discharge them earlier. The length of stay per admission fell. Hospitals also became concerned with physician practice behavior that increased the hospital's costs of care.

During the early 1980s important events were also occurring in the private sector. The new decade started with a recession, and as the United States began to recover, the dollar was very strong relative to other currencies. To survive the recession and to remain competitive internationally, business looked to reductions in their labor costs. Since health insurance was the fastest-growing labor expense, business began to pressure health insurers to better control both the use and cost of medical services. Competitive pressures forced insurers to increase the efficiency of the benefit package (including lower-cost substitutes to inpatient care such as outpatient surgery) by increasing patient price sensitivity (increasing deductibles and copayments) by and limiting use of the hospital (requiring the patient to receive prior authorization before being admitted to the hospital and then reviewing the patient's length of stay once in the hospital). These actions greatly reduced hospital admission rates and lengths of stay. Between 1970 and 1990, admissions per 1,000 population in Blue Cross plans declined 29 percent, from 127 per 1,000 to 90 per 1,000.

As a result of the federal DRG payment system, the above private programs, and a shift to the outpatient sector facilitated by changes in technology (both anesthetic and surgical techniques), hospital occupancy rates declined from 76 percent in 1980 to 66 percent in 1993. Hospitals had excess capacity. At the same time, increases in the supply of physicians created downward pressures on fees.

The preconditions for price competition were in place: there was excess capacity among suppliers, and demanders were interested in reducing their employees' medical expenses. The last necessary condition for price competition occurred in 1982 when the U.S. Supreme Court upheld the applicability of the antitrust laws to the medical sector. Successful antitrust cases were brought against the American Medical Association for their restrictions on advertising, against a medical society who threatened to boycott an insurer over physician fee increases, against a dental organization that boycotted an insurer's cost-containment program, against medical staffs that denied hospital privileges to physicians because they belonged to a health maintenance organization, and against hospitals whose mergers threatened to lessen price competition in their communities.

The applicability of the antitrust laws, excess capacity among providers, and business's and insurers' interest in lowering medical costs brought about profound changes in the medical marketplace. Traditional insurance plans lost market share as managed care plans, which control utilization and limit access to hospitals and physicians, grew. Preferred provider organizations (PPOs) were formed which included only physicians and hospitals that were willing to discount their prices. Employees and their families were offered price incentives in the form of lower out-of-pocket payments to use these less-expensive providers. Large employers and health insurers began to select PPO providers based on their prices, use of services, as well as on the outcomes of their treatment.

Although the federal government agreed to pay HMOs a capitated amount for enrolling Medicare patients in the mid-1980s, less than 10 percent of the aged voluntarily participated. In 1992 the federal government also changed the method of paying physicians under Medicare. A national fee schedule was adopted and volume-expenditure limits were established to limit the total rise in physician Medicare payments. Thus the main approach used by the federal government to contain Medicare expenditures continues to be the use of price controls and expenditure limits on payments to hospitals and physicians for services provided to Medicare patients.

The 1980s brought about a disruption in the traditional physician-patient relationship. Insurers use utilization review to control patient demand, emphasize outcomes and appropriateness of care, limit the patient's access to higher-priced providers, use case management for catastrophic illnesses, substitute less-expensive settings for more costly inpatient care, and provide price and other information to the employee when choosing a health plan. A variety of health plans now compete for enrollees on the basis of their premiums, benefits, patient out-of-pocket payments, and access to providers.

The use of cost-containment programs and the shift to outpatient care has lowered hospital occupancy rates. The increasing supply of physicians, particularly specialists, has left them with excess capacity. Both hospitals and physicians are now subject to intense competitive pressures, and these pressures are unlikely to change in the years ahead.

The Future

The pressures increasing demand, however, will continue to cause medical expenditures to increase for the forseeable future. New technology is believed to be the most important force behind rising expenditures. For example, the number of aged men having coronary artery bypass surgery increased from 1 per 400 in 1980 to 1 in every 100 in 1990; with regard to new equipment, the number of hospitals with magnetic resonance imagery (MRI) equipment increased by 500 percent between 1984 and 1991. As the population ages and as technological advances improve early diagnosis and new methods of treatment become available, there will be increased demand for medical services. The costs of providing medical services will also increase as more highly trained medical personnel are needed to handle the increased technology and as wage rates increase so as to attract more nurses and technicians to the medical sector. Thus even though the medical sector has become more efficient and price competitive, increased demands and higher costs of providing medical services will force medical expenditures higher.

Any method that arbitrarily seeks to reduce the rate of increase in medical expenditures will have to result in reduced access to both medical care and to new technology.

Choices to Make

Although this country spends more on health care than any other country, there is still a scarcity of funds to provide for all of our medical needs and all our population groups, such as the uninsured and those on Medicaid. Thus choices must be made. The first choice that we as a society must make is, How much of our scarce resources should be spent on medical care? What approach should be used for making this choice? Should the decision be left to individuals to determine how much of their incomes they want to spend on health care? Or should the government decide on the percent of GNP that goes to health care?

The second choice that must be made is, What is the best way of providing medical services? Would competition among health plans, or government regulation and price controls, achieve greater efficiency in the provision of medical services?

Third, how rapidly should medical innovation be introduced? Should regulatory agencies evaluate each medical advance and determine whether their benefits exceed their costs, or should the evaluation of those costs and benefits be left to the separate health plans competing for enrollees?

Fourth, how much should be spent on those who are medically indigent and how should their care be provided? Should the medically indigent be enrolled in a separate medical system, such as Medicaid, or should they be provided with vouchers to enroll in competing health plans?

These choices can be better understood when we are better aware of the consequences of each approach to deciding these choices, such as which groups benefit and which groups bear the costs. Economics clarifies the implications of different approaches to making these choices.

Reference

Letsch, S. W. "National Health Care Spending in 1991." *Health Affairs* 12 (Spring 1993): 94–110.

2

How Much Should We Spend on Medical Care?

The United States spends a greater portion of its GNP on medical care than does any other country. We are approaching 15 percent of GNP, and it is estimated that we will exceed 18 percent by the end of this decade. Can we afford to spend that much of our scarce resources on medical care? Why do we view growth in expenditures in other areas, such as automobiles, so much more favorably than expenditures on medical services? Increased medical expenditures create new health care jobs, do not pollute the air, save rather than destroy lives, and alleviate pain and suffering. More directly than any other industry, the medical sector serves those who are sick. Why shouldn't society be pleased that more resources are flowing into a sector that cares for the aged and the sick? It would seem to be a more appropriate use of a society's resources than spending those same funds on faster cars, alcohol, or other consumption items. And yet, increased expenditures on these other industries do not cause the concern that arises when medical expenditures increase.

Is the concern over rising medical costs merely the belief that we are not receiving value for our money, namely, that the additional medical services and technologies are not worth what it costs in relation to other uses of those resources? Or is there a more fundamental difference of opinion regarding the proper rate of increase in medical expenditures?

To understand why increased expenditures on medical services are a cause for concern, it is necessary to discuss what is an "appropriate" or "right" amount of expenditures. Only then can we evaluate whether we are spending "too much" on medical care. Further, if it is determined that too much is being spent, then we would have greater understanding as to the types of public policy necessary to achieve the "right" expenditure level.

Consumer Sovereignty

The "right" amount of health expenditures is based on a set of values and on the concept of economic efficiency. Given the limited resources available to us, these resources should be directed to their highest-valued uses, *as perceived by consumers*. Consumers decide how much to purchase based on their perception of the value they expect to receive and on how much they have to pay for it, knowing that an expenditure on one good means forgoing other goods and services. Consumers differ greatly on the value they place on medical care and on how much they are willing to forgo of other goods and services to spend more on health care. In a competitive market, consumers receive the full benefits of their purchases and in turn pay the full costs of receiving those benefits. When the benefits received from the last unit equal the cost of consuming that last unit, then the quantity consumed is said to be "optimal." If more or fewer services were consumed, the benefits received would be either less or greater than the cost of that service.

Consumer sovereignty can best be achieved in a competitive market system, which is able to accommodate consumers who have different values with regard to medical services and also differ on their willingness to pay for those services. Through their expenditures, consumers communicate their values in terms of the goods and services they wish to consume. Producers are directed by these expenditures to use the scarce resources to produce the goods desired by consumers. If producers are to survive and profit in competitive markets, they must be efficient in their use of resources and produce the goods consumers are willing to pay for; otherwise, they will be replaced by more efficient and responsive producers.

Some people believe, however, that consumer sovereignty should not be the basis for how much is spent on medical care. More than in other areas, patients lack information and have limited ability to judge needs for medical treatment. There is also the concern about the quality of care patients receive and how much care is appropriate.

Unfortunately, there is no perfect alternative. At one extreme, if medical care were free to all and physicians were to decide on the quantity of medical care, the result would be "too much" care. Physicians are likely to prescribe services as long as there is some perceived benefit, no matter how small, particularly since the physician would not be responsible for the cost of that care. The inevitable consequence of a free medical system is that the government then imposes an expenditure limit. Although physicians would still be responsible for determining who would receive care and for which diagnoses, it is likely "too little" care would then be provided; this is what occurs in government-controlled health systems, such as in Canada and Great Britain. Queues are established to ration the available medical care, and waiting times and age become criteria used for allocating the available medical resources.

No government that funds health care spends sufficient resources to provide all the care that is demanded at the going price. As does an individual making purchases, the government also makes trade-offs between the benefits received from additional health expenditures and the cost of those expenditures. However, the benefits and costs to the government are different than those used by consumers in their decision-making process. The benefits to the government represent the additional political support gained by further health expenditures; the cost is the lost political support of having to raise taxes to fund these programs or of shifting funds from other, politically popular, programs.

Let us therefore assume that the principle of consumer sovereignty will continue to be the guiding principle regarding how much is spent on medical expenditures. This does not mean, however, that this country is currently spending the "right" amount on medical services. To understand this, it is necessary to discuss the concept of economic efficiency.

Economic Efficiency

In the Provision of Medical Services

If medical services were produced in an inefficient manner, then medical expenditures would be excessive; for example, rather than treating a patient for ten days in the hospital, it might be possible to provide that medical treatment using fewer hospital days and a number of visits in the patient's home by a visiting nurse, with the same level of patient satisfaction and treatment outcome. Similarly, a treatment might be provided in an outpatient setting rather than in the hospital. Unless there are appropriate incentives for the providers of medical services to be efficient, it is unlikely that economic efficiency in the provision of medical services will be achieved.

Previously, when hospitals were paid on a cost-plus basis, their incentive was to increase their costs. Since the early 1980s, both the government and private sector have been pressuring for increased efficiency of the delivery system. Cost-based payment for hospitals has given way to payment based on fixed prices (DRGs). Price competition among hospitals and physicians has increased as insurance companies are themselves competing on the basis of premiums in the sale of group health insurance. PPOs, HMOs, and managed care systems have increased their market share. Hospitalization rates have declined with the increase in utilization review mechanisms. And the trend toward case management of catastrophic illness and monitoring providers for appropriateness of care and medical outcomes is increasing.

Although few would contend that the provision of medical services is as efficient as it could be, the proportion of waste in the health system is becoming smaller over time. With the growth of cost containment and managed care, inefficiency has been declining rather than increasing. Even if drastic reductions were made in private health insurance administrative costs of 50 percent (saving $20 billion in 1991), drug companies profits were reduced by 50 percent ($6 billion), and all physician incomes were reduced by 25 percent ($22 billion), these savings of approximately $48 billion would only be a one-time savings and would still be less than one year's annual percent increase in total medical expenditures. Inefficiency in the provision of medical services is not the main cause for concern over the rise in medical expenditures.

In the Use of Medical Services

Inefficiencies in the use of medical services occur when individuals do not have to pay the full cost of their choices; they consume "too much" medical care since their use of services is based on the out-of-pocket price they pay and that price is less than the cost of producing the service. The consequence is that the cost of providing the service exceeds the benefit received by the patient from consuming additional units of the service. The resources devoted to the production of these additional services could be better used in producing other services, such as education, that provide greater benefits.

The effect of paying less than the full price of a service is easily visualized with respect to some other consumer product, such as automobiles. If the price to the consumer of automobiles were greatly reduced, they would purchase more automobiles (and more costly ones). Resources used to produce these additional automobiles must come from resources used to produce other goods. Lowering the price the person has to pay results in increased use of medical services also. Studies have shown that patients who pay less out-of-pocket have more hospital admissions, physician visits, and use of outpatient services than patients who pay higher prices (Manning et al. 1987). This relationship between price and use of medical services also holds for patients classified by health status.

The reason use inefficiency is important in medical care is that the price of medical care has been *artificially* lowered to many consumers of medical services. The government subsidizes the purchase of medical care for both the poor and the aged under Medicaid and Medicare. Those who are eligible under these programs use more services than if they had to pay the full price themselves. Although the purpose of these programs was to increase their use of medical services, at times the artificially low prices result in inefficient use—for example, when the patient uses the more expensive emergency room rather than a physician's office in a nonemergent situation.

A greater concern with use inefficiency is with respect to the working population. Employer-purchased health insurance is not considered to be taxable income to employees. If the employer gave the same amount of funds directly to the employee in the form of higher wages, the employee would have to pay federal and state income tax as well as Social Security tax on that additional income. Since employer-purchased health insurance is not subject to these taxes, the purchase of health insurance, and hence additional medical services, is effectively subsidized by the government; employees do not pay the full cost of health insurance.

The greatest beneficiaries of this tax subsidy for the purchase of health insurance are those in higher-income tax brackets. For example, rather than receiving additional income as cash, which would then have been subject to high taxes (in the 1970s the highest federal income tax bracket was 70 percent), employees chose to have more of their increased wages paid in the form of increased health insurance coverage. Instead of spending after-tax dollars on vision and dental services, employees could purchase these services more cheaply when they were paid for with before-tax dollars in the form of health insurance.

"Too much" health insurance was purchased; the price of the insurance was reduced by the employee's tax bracket. Employees increased their health insurance since they did not have to pay the full cost of that coverage. As a consequence, the value of the additional insurance coverage was worth less to the employee than its full cost.

With the purchase of additional health insurance, the out-of-pocket price paid by the consumer for medical services declined; the result was an increase in use of all medical services covered by health insurance. As employees and their families became less concerned with the real cost of medical services, there were few constraints to limit the rise in medical expenditures. Had this "inefficiency" in use of medical services (as a result of the tax subsidy for the purchase of health insurance) been less, medical expenditures would have risen more slowly.

Inefficiencies in the use and in the provision of medical services are legitimate reasons for concern over how much is spent on medical care. Public policy should attempt to eliminate these government-caused inefficiencies. There are, however, other, less valid, reasons for concern over the rise in medical expenditures.

Government and Employer Concerns over Rising Medical Expenditures

The payers of medical expenditures, namely government and employers, are concerned over rising medical costs. Both the federal and state governments are large payers of medical expenditures. State governments pay one-half the costs of caring for the medically indigent in their states; the remaining half is paid for by the federal government. Medicaid expenditures are rising more rapidly than any other state expenditure and are causing states to reduce other politically popular programs; otherwise, the state would be forced to increase taxes. At the federal level, the government is also responsible for Medicare (acute medical services for the aged). The hospital portion of this program is financed by a specific Social Security tax, which has been increased numerous times, and the physician portion of the program (Part B) is financed from general income taxes. Expenditures under both of these programs have risen rapidly.

As shown in Table 2.1, federal health spending, as a proportion of total federal spending, is increasing rapidly, from 16.1 percent of total federal expenditures in 1992 to 23.6 percent in 1998. The federal government must control Medicare and Medicaid growth if it is to control the increase in federal expenditures.

Thus, even if there were no inefficiencies in the use or provision of medical services, increases in Medicare and Medicaid expenditures

Table 2.1 Federal Spending on Health, Fiscal Years 1965–1998 (billions of dollars)

	1965	1970	1975	1980	1985	1990	1992	1995	1998
Total federal spending	118.2	195.6	332.3	590.9	946.3	1,251.7	1,381.9	1,574.5	1,839.1
Federal health spending	3.1	13.9	29.5	61.8	108.9	168.0	222.7	320.2	434.2
Medicare	n.a.	6.2	12.9	32.1	65.8	98.1	119.0	171.7	239.3
Medicaid	0.3	2.7	6.8	14.0	22.7	41.1	67.8	105.0	145.9
Veterans Affairs	1.3	1.8	3.7	6.5	9.5	12.1	14.1	16.2	18.0
Other	1.5	3.2	6.1	9.2	10.9	16.6	21.8	27.3	31.0
Federal health spending as a percentage of total federal spending	2.6	7.1	8.9	10.5	11.5	13.4	16.1	20.3	23.6

Notes: Medicare expenditures are shown net of premium income from beneficiaries. "Other" includes federal employee and annuitant health benefits, as well as other health services and research. "Federal health spending" excludes spending for the military's CHAMPUS program.
Source: U.S. Congressional Budget Office (Washington, DC), calculations and projections, January 1993.

would still exceed what the government is willing to finance. If the government were the purchaser of 40 percent of all automobiles, the government would also become concerned with the price, use, and expenditures on automobiles. The pressure on government to continue funding Medicaid and Medicare either through increased taxes or larger budget deficits is driving government to seek ways to limit medical expenditure increases.

Similarly, unions and their employers are concerned with the rise in employee medical expenditures for reasons other than inefficiencies in the provision or in the use of services. As shown in Figure 2.1, business's spending on health insurance premiums has risen rapidly over time, both as a percent of total employee compensation and as a percent of business profits. Health insurance is part of an employee's total compensation. Employers are only interested in the total cost of their labor, not in the form the employee takes it, whether it is in wages or in health benefits. Thus the employee bears the cost of rising health insurance premiums because a rise in health insurance premiums results in lower cash wages. Large unions with generous health benefits want to reduce the rise in medical expenditures because they have seen more of their gains in compensation gone to finance their health insurance payments, rather than to increase employee wages.

Large employers have been seriously affected by the recent Financial Accounting Standards Board (FASB) ruling that employers who have promised medical benefits to their retirees are required to list this unfunded liability on their balance sheet. Employers have previously paid their retiree medical expenses only as they occurred and did not set aside funds as is done with pensions. By having to acknowledge these liabilities on their balance sheet, the net worth of many large corporations, such as the automobile companies, will decline by billions of dollars. Further, since these companies have to expense a portion of these future liabilities each year (not only for their present retirees but also for their future retirees), their earnings per share will decline. If the government were to reduce the rate of increase in medical expenditures, the net worth of companies with large unfunded retiree liabilities would be increased and their earnings per share would be higher.

It is important to be aware that there are different reasons for concern over rising medical expenditures. Whose concerns should drive public policy—the desire by government not to raise revenues to fund its share of medical services, union and employers' interest in lowering employee and retiree medical expenses, or society's desire to achieve

Figure 2.1   Business Spending on Health Premiums, 1965–1989

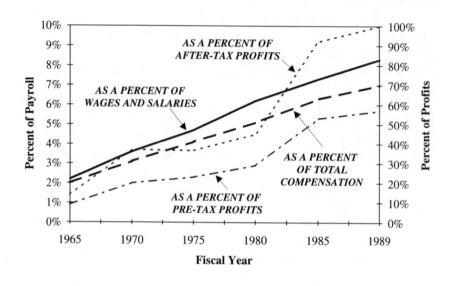

Source: R. Darman, Office of Management and Budget, and Executive Office of the President, *Introductory Statement: The Problem of Rising Health Costs*, 16 April 1991, p. 8.

the appropriate rate of increase in medical expenditures? The interests of government, unions, and large employers have little to do with achieving an appropriate rate of growth in medical expenditures. Instead, their own political and economic burdens are driving their proposals for limiting increases in medical expenditures.

Approaches to Limiting Increases
in Medical Expenditures

This country should strive to reduce inefficiencies in both the provision and the use of medical services. Inefficiencies in the provision of services are, however, becoming smaller as managed care plans reduce the cost of their plans so as to better compete for enrollees. Inefficiencies in the use of services is similarly declining as managed care plans attempt to control use of services by using utilization review, patient cost sharing, and capitation methods to pay physicians. As these inefficiencies are reduced, the growth in medical expenditures will approximate the "correct" rate of increase.

The public would naturally like to pay lower insurance premiums, less out-of-pocket for their medical care, and still have unlimited access to health care and to the latest in medical technology. But, as in other sectors of the economy, choices must be made.

The Clinton administration has proposed limiting the rise in health expenditures to the increase in inflation, population growth (about 1 percent per year), and productivity increases (about 1.6 percent per year). In other words, "real" per capita medical expenditures would increase, on average, by about 1.6 percent per year. Figure 2.2 shows the annual percent change in health expenditures and inflation since 1965. The annual percent change in total medical expenditures has, in almost all the years, exceeded the rate of inflation by more than 2½ percent (population and productivity growth). In the last several years alone, if this policy had been in effect, expenditures would have had to have been reduced by almost 4 percent annually.

Neither Canada nor Germany, two countries whose lower rates of increase in medical expenditures have been admired by many in the United States, have been able to sustain as low a rate of increase as has been proposed for this country. What are the consequences of such an approach?

The United States is undergoing important demographic changes; it is aging, and as it does so, the population requires more medical services, both for relief of suffering and for cures from its illnesses. Further, the most important reason for the rapid rise in medical expenditures has been the tremendous advances in medical science. Previously incurable diseases can now be cured, other diseases can be diagnosed at an earlier stage, and for others, even though no cure is available, life can be prolonged, such as with expensive drugs for AIDS patients. Limiting the growth in medical expenditures to the arbitrarily low rate that has been proposed will decrease investment in new technologies and limit the availability of medical services.

Cost-containment methods are currently available that can achieve some reduction in the rate of increase in medical expenditures; these would require either higher out-of-pocket payments or, through the use of managed care organizations, restricting enrollees to use only participating physicians and receiving approval before seeing a specialist. The middle class, however, is as yet unwilling to even make these trade-offs; they want both lower expenditures and unlimited access. And yet, to really

Figure 2.2 Annual Percent Growth in National Health Expenditures and the Consumer Price Index, 1965–1991

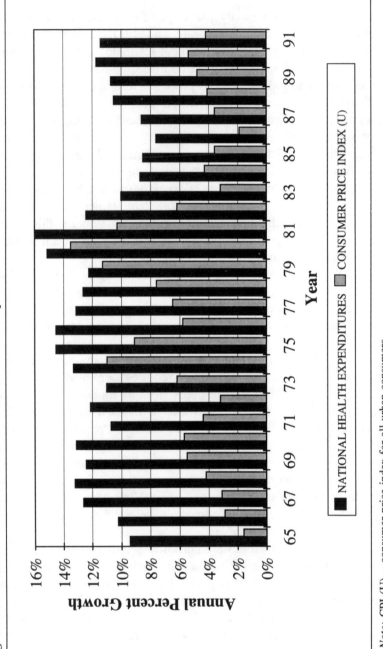

Note: CPI (U) = consumer price index for all urban consumers.
Sources: Data from U.S. Bureau of the Census, *Statistical Abstract of the Unites States, 1992,* and Organization for Economic Cooperation and Development, *OECD Health Systems,* Vol. I.

lower the rate of increase in expenditures and provide universal access to all will require more than just the cost-containment measures mentioned. Services and technology will have to become less available to many (Fuchs 1993).

Some politicians have, unfortunately, led the public to believe that it is not necessary to make these trade-offs; they claim that by eliminating waste in the health system, universal coverage can be achieved and everyone can have all the medical care they need, and at a lower cost. Such rhetoric merely postpones the time when the public realizes it must make the unpleasant choice between spending and access to care.

However, once the public understands that a trade-off must be made, then they are likely to want to make their own choices on how much of their resources should be spent on medical care, rather than having government or employer self-interest determine the rate of increase in medical expenditures. After all, who is better able to decide on issues of access and technology, and what those are worth, than the individuals who benefit and must pay for those services?

References

Fuchs, V. R. "No Pain, No Gain—Perspectives on Cost Containment." *The Journal of the American Medical Association* 269 (3 February 1993): 631–33.
Manning, W. G., J. P. Newhouse, N. Duan, E. B. Keeler, A. Leibowitz, and S. Marquis. "Health Insurance and the Demand for Medical Care: Evidence from a Random Experiment." *American Economic Review* 77 (June 1987): 251–77.

3

Do More Medical Expenditures Produce Better Health?

The United States spends more per capita on medical services and devotes a larger percent of its GNP to medical care than other countries, and yet our health levels are not proportionately higher. In fact, many countries that have lower per capita medical expenditures than the United States also have lower infant mortality rates and higher life expectancy. Is our medical system less efficient at producing health than these other countries? Or are medical expenditures less important than other factors that affect health levels?

Medical Services versus Health

Medical services are often, mistakenly, considered to be synonymous with health. When policymakers talk of "health reform," they really mean reform of the financing and delivery of medical services. Medical services consist of diagnosis and treatment of illness, which can lead to an increase in health. But medical services also consist of amelioration of pain and discomfort, reassurance to the worried well, and heroic treatments to those who are terminally ill. For example, more than 30 percent of all medical expenditures, almost $300 billion, are spent on just 1 percent of the population.[1] Increased medical expenditures, therefore, may have relatively little effect on our health levels.

The United States is generally acknowledged to have a technically superior medical system for treating acute illness (for a brief, but excellent, discussion of criteria to be used for evaluating a country's health

24

system, see Fuchs 1992). Financing and payment incentives have all been directed toward this goal. The training of physicians has emphasized treatment rather than prevention of illness. Public policy with regard to medical services has been concerned with two issues: (1) equity, namely, whether everyone has access to medical services and how those services should be financed, and (2) efficiency, such as whether medical services are efficiently produced. How to produce a medical treatment more efficiently, however, is not the same as knowing how to produce health efficiently.

Health policy, however, has been less well defined. The goal of health policy, presumably, should be an increase in health levels, or increased life expectancy, in which case we should be concerned with the most efficient ways to increase health levels. Once the policy objective becomes focused on health and its efficient production, then it is obvious that devoting increased resources to medical care is just one way to increase health, and it is unlikely to be the most efficient way to do so.

The more accurate the definition of health, the more difficult it is to measure. Health is a state of physical, mental, and social well-being. More simply, health is defined as the absence of disease or injury. Empirically, negative definitions are used to measure health, such as mortality rates and days lost due to sickness, or life expectancy. Definitions of health can be broad, such as the use of age-adjusted mortality rates, or they can be disease-specific, such as neonatal infant mortality rates (within the first 27 days of birth) and age-adjusted death rates from heart disease. The advantage of using such relatively crude measures is that they are readily available and are probably correlated with more comprehensive definitions of health. It should, however, be remembered that because measures of morbidity or quality of life are unavailable, it does not mean that they are unimportant or should be neglected in any analysis.

Health Production Function

To determine the relative importance of medical expenditures in decreasing mortality rates, economists have used the concept of a *health production function*. Simply stated, a health production function examines the relative contribution of each of the various factors that affect health so as to determine which is the most cost-effective way to improve health. For example, mortality rates are affected by the use of medical services, environmental conditions (such as the amount of air and water pollution), educational levels (which may indicate knowledge of prevention and ability to use the medical system when needed), and by lifestyle behavior (such as smoking, alcohol and substance abuse, and diet).

Each of these determinants of health have differential effects. For example, medical expenditures may initially cause a large decrease in mortality rates, as when a hospital is the first to establish an intensive care unit (ICU) in its community. But as additional ICUs are added within that community, the decline in mortality rate will become smaller. The first patients admitted to the ICU beds will be those most likely to benefit from the continuous monitoring of their condition. With a larger number of ICU beds, the beds may be either unused or the patients admitted to those beds will not be as critically ill. The investment in additional ICU beds will have less of an effect on patient mortality.

Figure 3.1 illustrates the relationship between increased medical expenditures and improvements in health levels. As expenditures are increased, there is a curvilinear, rather than a constant, effect on improved health. The "marginal" (additional) change on health becomes smaller as more is spent on that particular program. As shown in Figure 3.1, an initial expenditure to improve health, moving from A to B, has a much larger marginal benefit (effect) than subsequent investments, such as moving from C to D. The increase from H_1 to H_2 is greater than the increase from H_3 to H_4.

This same curvilinear relationship holds for each of the other determinants of health as well. Expenditures to decrease air pollution, such as mandating smog control devices on automobiles, will reduce the incidence of respiratory illness. Additional spending by automobile owners, such as having their smog control devices tested once a year rather than every three years to determine whether the devices are working properly, will further reduce air pollution. But the reduction in respiratory illness will not be as great as the initial expenditure to install smog control devices. The reduction in respiratory illness from additional expenditures to control air pollution gradually declines.

Everyone would probably agree that additional lives could be saved if more patients were admitted to ICUs (or respiratory illness decreased further with more frequent smog control inspections). There is always the possibility that more intensive monitoring might save a patient's life. However, those same funds could be spent on a prevention program to increase the number of women receiving mammograms, thereby diagnosing breast cancer earlier and increasing survival rates. The true "cost" of

Figure 3.1   The Effect of Increased Medical Expenditures on Health

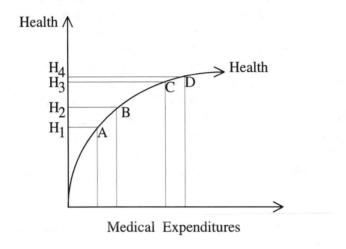

Medical Expenditures

any program to decrease mortality is the number of lives that could have been saved if those same funds were spent on another program.

Physicians, hospitals, dentists, and other health professionals all want increased government expenditures to decrease the unmet needs that they see among their populations. It would be impossible, however, for the government to spend all that is necessary to eliminate all medical, dental, mental, and other needs. To do so means forgoing the opportunity to eliminate other needs, such as exist in welfare and education, since resources are limited. At some point it becomes "too costly," in terms of forgone opportunities, to save all the lives that medical science is capable of achieving. Reallocating those same expenditures for apprehending drunk drivers or making highway improvements might save more lives.

Deciding which programs should be expanded to increase health levels requires a calculation of the cost per life saved for each of the programs that affect mortality rates. Based on the curve in Figure 3.1, assume that an additional medical expenditure of $1 million results in a movement from H_3 to H_4, or C to D, thereby saving 20 additional lives. The same $1 million spent on an educational program to reduce smoking may result in a movement from H_1 to H_2, or A to B, saving an additional 40 lives from lung cancer. The smoking reduction program therefore results in a lower cost per life saved ($1,000,000/40 = $25,000) than if those same funds were spent on additional medical services

($1,000,000/20 = $50,000). Continued expenditures on smoking cessation programs will result in a movement along the curve. After some point, fewer lung cancer deaths will be prevented, and lower cost per life saved could be achieved by spending additional funds on other programs, such as stronger enforcement of drunk driving laws.

Crucial to the calculation of cost per life saved is knowing, first, where the program, such as medical treatments or smoking cessation, is on the curve shown in Figure 3.1 and, second, what the cost is of expanding that program. The enormous and rapidly increasing medical expenditures in this country have most likely placed the return to medical services beyond point D. Further improvements in health levels from continued medical expenditures are very small. The cost of expanding medical treaments has also become very expensive.

Increasing Health Levels Cost-Effectively

Numerous empirical studies have found that further expenditures on medical services are not the most cost-effective way to increase health levels. Medical programs have a much higher cost per life saved than non-medical programs. Researchers have concluded that changing lifestyle behavior offers the greatest promise for lowering mortality rates, at a much lower cost per life saved.

The leading contributors to reductions in mortality rates over the past 25 years have been the decline in the neonatal infant mortality rate (infant deaths within the first 27 days of birth) and the reduction in deaths from heart disease.

Neonatal Infant Mortality Rate

The neonatal mortality rate represents three-fourths of the overall infant mortality rate; the decline in the overall mortality rate has been primarily due to the decline in the neonatal rate. From 1965 to 1990, the neonatal infant mortality rate declined an average of 2.6 percent per year. The neonatal mortality rates for Whites declined from 16.1 per 1,000 live births to 5.2 in 1990, as shown in Figure 3.2. For Blacks the decline was from 25.4 to 11.3. During that time period the availability of neonatal intensive care units increased, government subsidies were provided for family planning services for low-income women, maternal and infant nutrition programs expanded, Medicaid was initiated and paid for obstetric services for those with low incomes, and abortion was legalized.

One study found that, among Whites, increased educational levels and subsidized nutritional programs were most important in reducing the neonatal mortality rate. The availability of abortion, followed by the availability of neonatal ICUs, and the increase in education were most important among Blacks.

Knowing the reasons for the decline in neonatal mortality is insufficient, by itself, for deciding how to spend money to reduce neonatal mortality. For that it is important to know which are the more cost-effective programs. Joyce, Corman, and Grossman (1988) determined that the number of lives saved per 1,000 additional participants in teenage family planning programs, neonatal ICUs, and prenatal care were 0.6, 2.8, and 4.5, respectively. The costs of adding an additional 1,000 participants to each of these programs (in 1984 dollars) were $122,000, $13,616,000, and $176,000. To determine the cost per life saved from expanding each of these programs, the cost of the program was divided by the number of lives saved. As shown in Table 3.1, the cost per life saved

Figure 3.2 Neonatal Mortality Rates by Race, 1950–1990

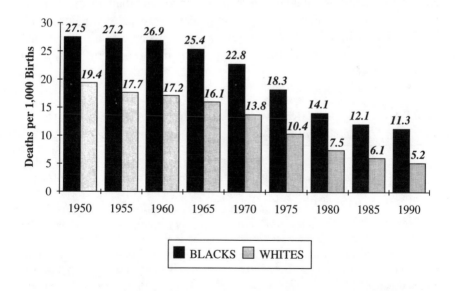

Sources: U.S. Department of Commerce, Bureau of the Census, (Washington, DC), *Historical Statistics of the United States, 1975,* and *Statistical Abstract of the United States, 1992.*

was $203,000 (which is determined by $122,000/0.6) for teenage family planning, $4,778,000 for neonatal ICUs, and $39,000 for prenatal care. The most cost-effective program for reducing neonatal mortality was prenatal care.

Reducing the potential number of women in high-risk pregnancies and the number of unwanted births (for example, by providing teenage family planning programs and prenatal care) offers a greater possibility of more favorable birth outcomes than by investing in additional neonatal ICUs.

Heart Disease Mortality Rate

The other leading contributor to the decline in mortality rates is the decline in coronary heart disease, which fell by 50 percent over the last 25 years. Contributing to this decline in mortality from heart disease have been improvements in medical technology (such as coronary by-pass surgery and coronary care units) as well as changes in lifestyle (such as the reduction in smoking, increased exercise, and changes in diet, which lowered cholesterol levels). Goldman and Cook (1984) concluded that lifestyle changes were more important than medical interventions and were also much less expensive (see also McGinnis and Foege 1993). These lifestyle changes, however, were not uniform among the population; they were more likely to be undertaken by those with more education.

Table 3.1   Cost per Life Saved among Three Programs to Reduce Neonatal Mortality

	Number of Lives Saved per 1,000 Additional Participants	Cost of Each Program per 1,000 Additional Participants	Cost per Life Saved ($1984 in thousands)
Teenage family planning	0.6	$ 122,000	$ 203,000
Neonatal ICUs	2.8	13,616,000	4,778,000
Prenatal care	4.5	176,000	39,000

Reprinted with permission as it appeared in T. Joyce, H. Corman, and M. Grossman, "A Cost-Effectiveness Analysis of Strategies to Reduce Infant Mortality," *Medical Care* 26 (April): 348–60. © 1988 J. B. Lippincott Company.

Causes of Death by Age Group

Perhaps the clearest indication of the importance of lifestyle behavior as a determinant of mortality is the causes of death by age group. As shown in Table 3.2, the main causes of death for young adults are accidents (particularly auto), homicides, and suicides. For those in the middle-age groups, accidents, cancer, HIV infection, heart disease, suicides, and homicides are the major causes of death. And for those in late middle age, cancer and heart disease are the leading causes of death. After examining data by cause of death, Victor Fuchs concluded that medical services have a smaller effect on health than the way in which people live: " . . . the greatest potential for reducing coronary disease, cancer, and the other major killers still lies in altering personal behavior" (1974, 46).

Since expenditures on medical services have been shown to be less cost-effective in reducing mortality rates than are changes in lifestyle behavior, why does this country spend an increasing portion of its resources on medical care?

First, health insurance coverage has been so comprehensive, with low deductibles and small copayments, that individuals face a very low out-of-pocket price when they go to the hospital or to a specialist. Thus patients use more medical services than if they had to pay a greater portion of the cost. The expression "The insurance will cover it" is indicative of the lack of incentives facing patients and their providers. The public has also had little incentive to compare prices among different providers since the costs they would incur searching for less-expensive providers would exceed any savings on their already low copayments. It is also not surprising, given these low copayments and the incentives inherent in fee-for-service payments to providers, that enormous resources are spent on those in their last year of life. The consequence of this behavior has been rapidly rising medical expenditures and limited reductions in mortality rates.

Second, the primary objective of the government's medical expenditures has not been to improve health and decrease mortality rates. Medicare benefits the elderly; approximately one-half of Medicaid expenditures are for care of the elderly in nursing homes. The purpose of these government expenditures is to assist the aged in financing their medical needs. Had the government's objective been to increase the nation's health, the types of services financed would have been very different, as would be the age groups who would most benefit from those expenditures.

Table 3.2   Leading Causes of Death by Age Group, 1989

Age Group	Major Causes of Death	Deaths per 100,000
15–24	All causes	99.9
	Accidents	45.8
	Homicide	16.9
	Suicide	13.3
	Cancer	5.1
	Heart disease	2.6
	HIV infection	1.7
25–44	All causes	176.1
	Accidents	35.4
	Cancer	26.2
	HIV infection	20.3
	Heart disease	19.0
	Suicide	14.8
	Homicide	13.9
45–64	All causes	813.3
	Cancer	290.9
	Heart disease	241.5
	Stroke	32.5
	Accidents	32.4
	Pulmonary disease	28.0
	Liver disease/cirrhosis	24.7
	Diabetes	20.9

Source: U.S. Bureau of the Census (Washington, DC), *Statistical Abstract of the United States, 1992.*

Even though medical expenditures have a relatively small marginal effect on health, it would be incorrect to conclude that the government should limit all medical expenditure increases. To an individual, additional medical services may be worth their additional cost, even when they are not subsidized in their purchase of medical services. As incomes increase, people are willing to purchase medical services to relieve anxiety and seek relief of pain, which are not life-saving events. These are entirely appropriate personal expenditures. From the government's perspective, it is also appropriate to finance medical services for those with low incomes. As society becomes wealthier, individuals and government are willing to make more non–life-saving medical expenditures. These "consumption" as compared to "investment" type medical expenditures are appropriate, as long as they are recognized by all for what they are.

When government attempts to improve the health of those with low incomes, using the concept of a health production function will enable expenditures to be directed toward those programs that are most cost-effective, that is, result in the lowest cost per life saved. Allocating funds in this manner will achieve a greater reduction in mortality rates, for a given total expenditure, than any other allocation method.

The health production function concept is increasingly being used by employers and managed care organizations who face financial pressures to reduce their medical costs. Employer use of health risk appraisal questionnaires is a recognition that their employees' health can be improved, less expensively, by changes in lifestyle behavior. Incentives given to their employees to stop smoking, reduce their weight, and exercise enable employers to retain a skilled workforce longer, while reducing medical expenditures. The emphasis by managed care organizations on reducing per capita medical costs is leading several of them to identify their high-risk groups who can benefit from early intervention of preventive measures so as to reduce costly medical treatments.

The recognition by government, employers, managed care organizations, and individuals that resources are scarce and that their objective is improved health rather than provision of additional medical services will lead to new approaches to increase health. The concept of a health production function should clarify the trade-offs between different programs and improve the allocation of expenditures.

Note

1. Also, 58 percent of total medical expenditures were spent on 5 percent of the population. Nearly one-half of those upon whom a great amount of money was spent were elderly (Berk and Monheit 1992).

References

Berk, M., and A. Monheit. "The Concentration of Health Expenditures: An Update." *Health Affairs* 11 (Winter 1992): 145–49.

Fuchs, V. R. "The Best Health Care System in the World?" *Journal of the American Medical Association* 268 (19 August 1992): 916–17.

Fuchs, V. R. *Who Shall Live?* New York: Basic Books, 1974.

Goldman, L., and F. Cook. "The Decline in Ischemic Heart Disease Mortality Rates: An Analysis of the Comparative Effects of Medical Interventions and Changes in Lifestyle." *Annals of Internal Medicine* 101 (December 1984): 825–36.

Joyce, T., H. Corman, and M. Grossman. "A Cost-Effectiveness Analysis of Strategies to Reduce Infant Mortality." *Medical Care* 26 (April 1988): 348–60.

McGinnis, J. M., and W. H. Foege. "Actual Causes of Death in the United States." *Journal of the American Medical Association* 270 (10 November 1993): 2207–12.

4

In Whose Interest Does the Physician Act?

The physician has always played a crucial role in the delivery of medical services. Even though only 25 percent of total medical expenditures are for physician services, the physician controls the use of a much larger portion of total medical resources. In addition to their own services, physicians determine admission to the hospital, the length of stay once in the hospital, the use of ancillary services, referrals to specialists, and even the necessity for services in nonhospital settings, such as home care. Any public policies that affect the financing and delivery of medical services must consider the response by physicians to those policies. The physician's knowledge and motivation will affect the efficiency with which medical services are delivered.

The role of the physician has been shaped by two important characteristics of the medical system. The first is the legal system: only physicians are permitted to provide certain services. Second, both patients and insurers lack the necessary information to make many medical-related decisions. The patient depends upon the physician for the diagnosis and the recommended treatment and has limited information on the qualifications of the physician or the specialists to whom they are referred. This lack of information by patients on their diagnosis, required treatment, and quality of medical providers places the physician in a unique relationship to the patient. The physician becomes the patient's agent.

The Physician as a Perfect Agent for the Patient

A major controversy in the medical economics literature is with regard to the agency relationship. In whose best interest does the physician act? If the physician were a perfect agent for the patient, the physician would prescribe the mix of institutional settings and the amount of care in each, based on the patient's medical needs, ability to pay for medical services, and preferences. The physician would behave as would the patient, if the patient were as fully informed as the physician. Traditional indemnity insurance, which was the prevalent form of health insurance, reimbursed the physician fee-for-service; neither the physician nor the patient were fiscally responsible or at risk for use of the hospital and medical services.

Prior to the 1980s, Blue Cross coverage was predominately for hospital care. Even though it was more costly in terms of resources used, it was less expensive *for the patient* to receive a diagnostic workup in the hospital than as an outpatient. Even though this was an inefficient use of resources, the physician acted in the patient's and not the insurer's interest. Similarly, if a woman wanted to stay a few extra days in the hospital after giving birth, the physician would not discharge her before she was ready to return home.

As the patient's agent, the quantity and type of services that the physician prescribes would be based on the value of that additional care to the patient and the patient's cost for that care. As long as the value of that care to the patient exceeds the patient's costs for that care, the physician would prescribe it. By only considering the patient's costs and benefits of additional medical services, the costs to society of those resources and the costs to the insurance company were neglected.

Indemnity insurance and the role of the physician as the patient's agent led the physician to practice what Victor Fuchs (1968) referred to as the "technologic imperative." Regardless of how small the benefits were to the patient or how costly it was to the insurer, the physician would prescribe the best medical care that was technically possible. As a consequence, heroic measures were provided to patients in the last few months of their lives and inpatient hospital costs rose rapidly. It was a rational economic decision to prescribe "low benefit" care since it still exceeded the patient's cost, which was virtually zero with insurance.

Supplier-Induced Demand

The view of the physician as the patient's agent, however, neglects the economic self-interest of the physician. As shown in Figure 4.1 large increases in both the total number of physicians and in the number of physicians relative to the population occurred throughout the 1970s and 1980s. The standard economic model, which assumes the physician is a perfect agent for the patient, would predict that an increase in supply, other things being equal, would result in a decline in physicians' fees, visits per physician, and, consequently, physician incomes.

Increases in the physician/population ratio, however, did not lead to declines in physician incomes. This observation led to the development of an alternative theory of physician behavior. Physicians are believed to behave differently when their own incomes are adversely affected. In addition to being the patient's agent, physicians are a supplier of a service. Their incomes depend upon how much of that service they supply. Do physicians use their information advantage over both patients and insurers to benefit themselves? This model of physician behavior is referred to as "supplier-induced demand" (for recent discussions of demand inducement, see McGuire and Pauly 1991; Pauly et al. 1992).

The supplier-induced demand theory assumes that if the physician's income falls, the physician will use their role as the patient's agent to

Figure 4.1　Number of Physicians and Physician-Population Ratio, 1950–1990

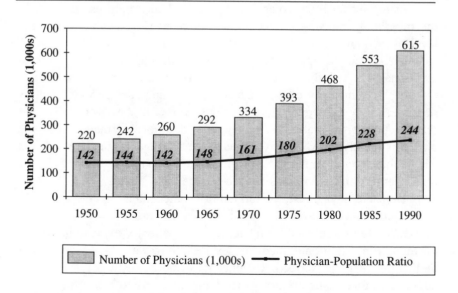

Source: American Medical Association (Chicago, IL), *Physician Characteristics and Distribution, 1992.*

prescribe additional services. The physician provides the patient with misinformation so as to increase the patient's demand for physician services, thereby increasing the physician's income.

Physicians might rationalize some demand inducement in that additional services or tests would be beneficial to the patient. However, as more and more services are recommended, the physician must choose between the additional income received versus the psychological cost of knowing that those additional services are not really necessary. At some point the additional revenue the physician receives is not worth the psychological cost of prescribing such services. The physician must make a trade-off between increased income and the dissatisfaction the physician receives from knowingly providing too many services. The idea that physicians induce demand only to the extent that they can maintain or achieve a given level of income is referred to as the "target income" theory.

Thus one might envisage a spectrum of demand inducement, depending upon the pyschological cost to the physician of greater demand inducement. At one end of the spectrum, there are those physicians who act solely in their patient's interest; they do not induce demand to increase or even maintain their incomes. At the other end of the spectrum are physicians who attempt to increase their incomes by inducing demand as much as possible; this latter group of physicians presumably incurs little psychological cost when it induces demand. In the middle are physicians who induce demand to achieve some target level of income.

The extent to which the physician is willing and able to induce additional demand for medical services is controversial. Few believe that the large majority of physicians would induce demand as much as possible, solely to increase their incomes. Similarly, few would disagree that the physician is able to induce some additional demand. Thus the choice is mainly between physicians as perfect agents for their patients versus the target income model of physician behavior. The issue is, How much demand are physicians able to induce?

Demand inducement is limited to some extent by the patient's recognition that the additional medical benefits are not worth the time or cost of returning to the physician. The patient's evaluation of the benefits from additional medical services, however, varies according to the treatment prescribed. Patients may more easily determine that additional office visits are not worth their time and cost of returning. It is, however, more difficult for the patient to evaluate the benefits from certain surgical services. Thus demand inducement is more likely to occur for those services for which the patient is most ignorant.

Many studies have attempted to determine the extent of demand inducement (see Feldstein 1993, 86–90, 187–91). This issue is still unresolved. There is evidence that the larger the supply of physicians (in relation to the population), the higher is the use of physician services. This relationship, however, may merely indicate that physicians locate where the population has higher insurance coverage and, consequently, a greater demand for their services. One study concluded that primary care physicians are limited in the amount of demand they can induce, although it is not known how much demand they may have already induced. The positive correlation between the number of surgeons and the number of surgeries has been used as empirical support for the supplier-induced demand theory. Further, studies have found that the rate of surgeries for such procedures as tonsillectomies and hysterectomies to be higher when physicians were paid fee-for-service than when physicians had different income incentives, such as being part of a health maintenance organization. It appears that demand inducement is more of a concern with surgeries because patients are less well informed about whether they need the surgery.

Increase in Physician Supply

The large increase in physician supply since the 1960s serves to illustrate the importance of knowing which model of physician behavior, the "perfect agent" or "supplier-induced demand," is more prevalent. As a perfect agent for the patient, the physician would continue to consider only the patient's medical and economic interests when prescribing a treatment, regardless of the fact that their incomes may decline because the greater supply of physicians may decrease the number of patients in their practice.

According to the supplier-induced demand model, an increase in the supply of physicians will cause physicians to induce demand to prevent their incomes from falling. Total medical expenditures would also increase as a larger number of physicians, each with fewer patients, attempt to maintain their incomes. Thus, depending upon whether one believes in standard economic models or supplier-induced demand, increases in the supply of physicians lead to quite opposite predictions as to its effect on physician visits, prices, and incomes.

Insurer's Response to Demand Inducement

Insurers recognize that under fee-for-service payment the physician acts as either the patient's agent or to maintain their own income. In either case, the value of additional benefits is lower than the insurer's cost of those services. Consequently, the premium for indemnity insurance will be higher than for HMOs, which will cause more of the insurer's subscribers to switch to HMOs. In recent years, therefore, insurers have developed mechanisms to overcome the information advantage that the physician has over both the insurer and the patient to serve either the patient's or the physician's interests.

Insurers have, for example, implemented second opinions for surgery. Once a physician recommends certain types of surgery whose medical necessity is doubtful, such as back surgery, the patient may be required to receive a second opinion from a list of physicians approved by the insurer. Another approach used by insurers is the creation of preferred provider organizations. Physicians are selected based on whether they offer lower fees, use fewer medical services, and are considered to be of high quality. A third approach is to use utilization review. Prior to a hospital admission a patient must receive the insurer's approval; otherwise, the patient is subject to a financial penalty. The length of stay in the hospital may also be subject to approval.

These cost-containment approaches by insurers are an attempt to address the imbalances in physician and patient incentives under fee-for-service, and to ensure that the patient receives appropriate care (when the physician acts to increase his or her own income) and that the resource costs of treatment are considered along with their expected benefits.

HMOs

The growth of HMOs and capitation payment provides physicians with incentives to increase their incomes opposite from those of traditional indemnity fee-for-service. HMOs typically reward their physicians with profit-sharing or bonuses if their enrollees' medical costs are *lower* than their annual capitation payments. What are the likely effects on an HMO's patients of these differing models of physician behavior, the "perfect agent" and the "imperfect agent," one who is interested in increasing income, possibly at the patient's expense?

A perfect agent type of physician would continue to provide the patient in an HMO setting with appropriate medical services. Regardless of the effect of profit-sharing on their income or pressures from the HMO to reduce use of services, the perfect agent physician would be primarily concerned with protecting the patient's interest and providing him or her with the best medical care. There would be little likelihood of underservice. And, unlike indemnity insurance, within an HMO the physician would not need to be concerned over whether the patient's insurance covered the medical cost in different settings. There are also fewer deductibles and copayments for HMO patients. Thus the settings chosen for providing the patient's treatment are likely to be less costly for both the patient and the HMO.

The concern that patients would be underserved in an HMO is with regard to "imperfect agent" physicians, those who attempt to increase their incomes. HMO physicians have an incentive to provide fewer services to their patients and to serve a larger number of patients. HMO physicians who are concerned with the size of their incomes are more likely to respond to the profit-sharing incentives. At times a physician, who may even be salaried, may succumb to an HMO's pressures to reduce use of services and thereby become an imperfect agent. Underservice becomes a concern for HMO patients. If HMO patients believe they are being denied timely access to the physician, specialist services, or to needed technology, they are likely to either try and switch HMO physicians or disenroll at the next open enrollment period. Too high a rate of dissatisfaction with certain HMO physicians could be an indication of underservice.

An HMO should also be concerned with underservice by its physicians. Although the HMO's profitability will increase if its physicians provide too few services, an HMO that limits access to care and fails to satisfy its subscribers risks losing market share.

The more knowledgeable subscribers are on access to care provided by different HMOs, the greater will be the HMO's financial incentive not to pressure their physicians to underserve their patients and to actually monitor their physicians to guard against underservice. Although it is costly in both time and money for individuals to gather information on HMOs and their physicians on how well their enrollees are served, it is less costly for employers to gather this information, make it available to their employees, and even limit the HMOs from which their employees can choose.

Informed Purchasers

Informed purchasers are necessary if the market is to discipline imperfect agents, who may be the HMO itself or its physicians. An HMO's reputation is a costly asset that can be reduced by "imperfect agent" type physicians underserving their patients. Performance information and competition among HMOs for informed purchasers should prevent these organizations from underserving their enrollees. The financial, reputational, and legal costs of underservice should mitigate the financial incentives to underprescribe in an HMO.

Both indemnity insurers and HMOs lack information on the patient's diagnosis and appropriate treatment needs. Thus the insurer's (and HMO's) profitability depends upon the physician's knowledge and treatment recommendations. Depending upon the type of insurance plan and the incentives physicians face, there is a potential inefficiency in the provision of medical services. Physicians may prescribe either too many or too few services. When "too many" services are prescribed, the value of those additional services to the patient may not be worth the costs of producing them. "Too few" services are also inefficient in that patients may not realize that the value of the services and technology they did not receive are greater than their physician led them to believe and for which they were willing to pay. To decrease the inefficiencies arising from "too many" services as a result of demand inducement, indemnity insurers who pay fee-for-service have instituted cost-containment methods.

Medicare, as a fee-for-service insurer for physician services for the aged, has, however, not yet undertaken similar cost-containment methods to limit supplier-induced demand. Until Medicare is able to institute such mechanisms, target income physicians will continue to be able to manipulate the information they provide to the aged, change the visit coding to receive higher payment, and decrease the time spent per visit with aged patients.

Monitoring of physician behavior is increasing within HMOs and other capitated programs. Physicians who were previously in fee-for-service and increased their incomes by prescribing too many services are being reviewed to ensure they understand the change in incentives. And once they are aware of the new incentives for increasing their incomes, imperfect agent physicians must be monitored to ensure that they do not underserve their HMO patients.

The market for medical services is changing. Insurers and large employers are attempting to overcome the physician's information advantage by profiling physicians according to their prices, use and appropriateness of services provided, and their treatment outcomes. As this occurs, there will be less opportunity for target income physicians to benefit themselves at the expense of the insurer. Demand inducement, to the extent it exists, will diminish. Hopefully, with improved monitoring systems and better measures of patient outcomes, physicians will behave as efficient agents, providing the "appropriate" quantity and quality of medical services, where the costs as well as the benefits of additional treatment are considered.

Not all insurers or employers, however, are engaged in these informational and cost-containment activities. Those who are not will still be at an informational disadvantage to the physician and the HMO. Insurers and employers who are less knowledgeable regarding the services provided to their employees will be paying for overuse of services and demand-inducing behavior by fee-for-service providers and underservice by HMO physicians. At some point such purchasers will realize it is worthwhile to invest in greater information that will lower their medical expenditures and improve the quality of care provided.

Summary

Under fee-for-service payment, the inability of patients and their insurers to distinguish between target income and perfect agent physicians led to the growth of cost-containment methods. Changes that are occurring in the private sector and in government physician payment systems must consider that there are different types of physicians and, unless appropriately monitored, the response by imperfect agent physicians will make it difficult to achieve the intended objectives.

References

Feldstein, P. J. *Health Care Economics.* Albany, NY: Delmar Publishers Inc., 1993.

Fuchs, V. R. "The Growing Demand for Medical Care." *The New England Journal of Medicine* 279 (25 July 1968): 190–95.

McGuire, T. G., and M. V. Pauly. "Physician Response to Fee Changes with Multiple Payers." *Journal of Health Economics* 10, no. 4 (1991): 385–410.

Pauly, M. V., J. M. Eisenberg, M. H. Radany, M. H. Erder, R. Feldman, and J. S. Schwartz. *Paying Physicians: Options for Controlling Cost, Volume, and Intensity of Services.* Ann Arbor, Michigan: Health Administration Press, 1992.

5

Rationing Medical Services

No country can afford to provide unlimited amounts of medical services to everyone. Although few would disagree that there is waste in the current system, even if that waste were eliminated and those resources redirected, all of this country's medical needs could not be fulfilled. There would be a large one-time savings from elimination of inefficiencies, but driven by population growth, an aging population, and advances in medical technology, medical expenditures would continue to increase at a rate faster than inflation. And as new experimental treatments, such as bone marrow transplants, are developed—no matter how uncertain or small their effect might be—making these routinely available to all those who might conceivably benefit would be very costly. The resources needed to eliminate all of our medical needs, including prescription drugs, mental health, long-term care, dental, and vision, as well as for services that are acute, chronic, and preventive, would be enormous.

The cost of eliminating all medical needs, no matter how small, means foregoing the benefits of spending those resources to meet other needs, such as on food, clothing, housing, and education. That is the real cost of fulfilling all of our medical needs. Since no country can afford to spend unlimited resources on medical services, each society must choose some mechanism to ration or to limit access to medical services.

Government Rationing

There are two methods by which "rationing" occurs. The first, and most frequently used definition, is when the government limits access to goods and services. In World War II, food, gasoline, and other goods were rationed; their prices were kept artificially low but people could not buy all they wanted at the prevailing price. Similarly, in the 1970s, a gasoline shortage developed when the government kept the price of gasoline below its market price. The available supply was "rationed" by having people wait long hours at gasoline stations, even though they were willing, but not permitted, to pay higher prices.

This type of rationing is also used to allocate medical services in various countries, such as Great Britain (Aaron and Schwartz 1990). The British government sets low prices for medical services and limits their expenditures. Since there is a shortage of services at their prevailing prices, these scarce services are allocated according to a person's age, such as denying kidney transplants to those over a certain age, or according to a queue, where a person may wait months or even years for certain surgical procedures.

In the United States, only the state of Oregon has proposed such an explicit system of rationing medical services. In contrast to other states that provide unlimited services to a small portion of those who are poor, the Oregon legislature decided to limit access to expensive procedures, such as organ transplants, to those on Medicaid and, in turn, to increase Medicaid eligibility to more low-income persons. The state ranked all medical services according to the outcomes that could be expected from treatment, such as "prevents death with full recovery," and according to their effect on the quality of life. Since the state budget is unlikely to ever be sufficient to fund all medical procedures to all of the poor, those procedures at the lower end of the rankings would not be funded.

Rationing by Ability to Pay

Among the general population in the United States, such explicit rationing of medical services is not used. Instead, a different type of "rationing" is used, namely, to distribute goods and services according to those who can afford to pay for them. There are no "shortages" of services for those who are willing to pay (either out-of-pocket or through insurance). Those with low incomes and without health insurance receive fewer medical services than those who have higher incomes.

Medical services involve a great deal of discretionary use. Empirical studies show that a 10 percent increase in income leads to an approximate 10 percent increase in medical expenditures. As incomes increase, the amounts spent on medical services increase proportionately. This relationship between income and medical spending exists not only in this country but across all countries. As shown in Figure 5.1, the higher the country's income, the greater its medical expenditures.

This observed relationship between income and medical expenditures suggests that as people become wealthier they prefer to spend more on medical services, to receive a greater quantity of services and higher-quality services by making greater use of specialists, and they are willing to pay more not to have to wait to receive those services.

Decision Making by Consumers of Medical Services

Understanding why people use medical services thus requires more than knowing whether or not they are ill. Also important are their attitudes

Figure 5.1   Health Spending and Personal Income in Different Countries, 1990

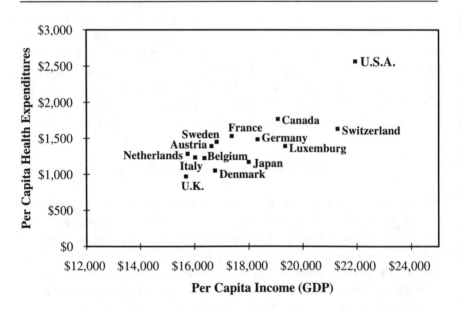

Note: All values are U.S. dollars measured in GDP purchasing power parities.
Source: Organization for Economic Cooperation and Development (Paris, France), *OECD Health Data File, 1992.*

toward seeking care, the prices they must pay for such care, and their incomes.

Whether or not rationing is based on ability to pay or on government limits on medical services, patients are faced with prices they must pay for medical services. These prices may be artificially low, as in Great Britain or Canada, or they may reflect the cost of providing those medical services, as in a market-oriented system. Regardless of how those prices are determined, they are an essential ingredient for consumer decision making.

Consumers spend (allocate) their money based upon the value they place on different needs, on how much income they have, and the prices of their different choices. The consumer is faced with an array of choices, each offering additional benefits, but each choice costs different amounts of money. Consumers choose, not just on the basis of the additional benefits they would receive, but also on the cost of achieving those benefits. It is in this manner that prices enable consumers to decide on which services to allocate their incomes. Making one choice means forgoing other choices. Similarly, as the prices of some choices increase while others decrease, consumers are likely to rearrange their purchases. An increase in their incomes allows consumers to buy more of everything.

The Marginal Benefit Curve

Figure 5.2 illustrates the relationship between use of services and the cost to the patient of those services. The marginal benefit curve shows that the additional (marginal) benefit the patient receives from additional visits declines as use of services increases. For example, a patient concerned about his or her health will benefit a great deal from the first physician visit. The physician will take the patient's history, perhaps perform some diagnostic tests, and possibly write a prescription for the patient. A follow-up visit will enable the physician to determine whether the diagnosis and treatment were appropriate and provide reassurance to the patient. The marginal benefit of that second visit will not be as high as the first visit. Additional return visits, without any indication of a continuing health problem, will provide further reassurance, but the value to the patient of those additional visits will be much lower than the initial visits.

How rapidly the marginal benefit curve declines depends upon the attitudes of the patient toward seeking care and the value they place on that additional care. Not all patients place the same value on medical

Figure 5.2   The Relationship between Prices, Visits, and Marginal
Benefit of an Additional Visit

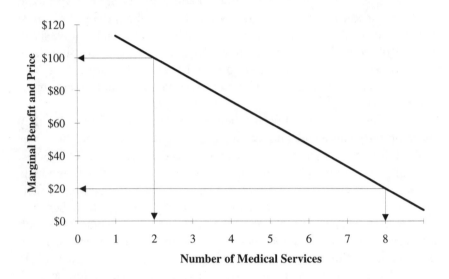

Number of Medical Services

services. For some, the marginal benefit curve will decline very quickly
after the initial treatment; for others it will be very gradual.

The actual number of patient visits is determined by the cost to the
patient of each visit. Given the patient's marginal benefit curve and a
price per visit of $100, as shown in Figure 5.2, the marginal benefit to
the patient of the first visit exceeds their cost of $100. The patient will
demand a total of two visits because the marginal benefit of that second
visit equals the cost of that visit. If the patient were to make more than
two visits, the value the patient receives from that additional (third) visit
would be less than its cost.

Thus the demand for medical services is determined by the value to
the patient (either real or imagined) of those visits and the patient's cost
of each visit. When the cost is greater than the value of an additional
visit, the patient would not make the additional visit; the patient could
receive greater value for his or her money by spending it on other goods
and services.

Health insurance reduces the cost of medical care to the patient.
While the physician (or hospital) is paid the full price by the insurer, the
patient pays a reduced out-of-pocket price. If the charge for a physician's
office visit is $100 and health insurance pays 80 percent of the charge,

then the "real" price to the patient is only $20. As the cost to the patient of an office visit declines from $100 to $20, the patient will increase the number of visits. The patient will make additional visits until the value received from that last visit is worth only $20.

The patient's decision to use medical services is based solely on a calculation of his or her own costs (copayment) and the perceived value of those additional visits. Although the real cost of each visit is $100, the cost to the patient of additional visits is only $20. The consequence is "too much" medical care—the value to the patient of additional visits is worth less than the full cost of those visits.

Travel and waiting costs are usually incurred by the patient in using medical services. The importance of these costs differs among patients. Typically, retired persons have low waiting costs, while working mothers have high waiting costs. To predict use of services, travel and waiting costs as well as out-of-pocket payments must be weighted against the marginal benefit of another visit. A medical system that has high out-of-pocket payments and low waiting costs will have a different effect on usage patterns than a system that relies on low prices but high waiting costs.

An important empirical question is, How rapid is the decline in value of additional services to the patient? If the first visit is worth more than $100 to the patient and the second visit is only worth $10, there will be little, if any, overuse of medical services. If, however, a second visit is worth $100, and the value of subsequent visits declines slowly, the patient will find it worthwhile to make many visits before the value of a visit falls below $20.

Price Sensitivity

Research on the relationship between the out-of-pocket price paid by the patient and use of medical services indicates that for some medical services the decline in value of additional services is gradual. For example, a 10 percent reduction in the price of mental health services would lead to a 10 percent increase in use of services. Physician and hospital services are less price sensitive; lowering prices by 10 percent would increase use by only 2 percent. Long-term care services are very price sensitive. A 10 percent reduction in nursing home prices would lead to a 20 percent increase in use. This finding suggests that if long-term care were included as part of national health insurance, there would be large increases in nursing home use and expenditures.

The price sensitivity faced by individual physicians, hospitals, and other providers is much greater since each provider is a possible substitute to other providers. For example, while a 10 percent overall price decrease leads to a 2 percent increase in overall use of physician services, if an individual physician raises (or lowers) his or her price by 10 percent, and other physicians do not change their prices, the individual physician will lose (or gain) large numbers of patients, approximately 30 percent. Similarly, there is greater price sensitivity toward any single health plan than to health insurance in general. When employees have a choice of health plans and have to pay an out-of-pocket premium (copremium) for these plans, the employees' choice of health plan is very price sensitive. One study found that a $5 increase in an HMO copremium, with the copremiums of other health plans unchanged, resulted in a 66 percent disenrollment (Long et al. 1988).

Moral Hazard

When patients use more medical services because their insurance covers 80 percent of the cost of those services, the insurance industry refers to this behavior as "moral hazard." This term means that having insurance changes a person's behavior; the cost of medical services to the insurance company is increased. Those with insurance (or more comprehensive insurance) use more services, see more specialists, and incur higher medical costs than those who do not have insurance (or less comprehensive insurance), and the value placed on many of these additional services by the patient and their physician are lower than their full costs.

Evidence from the RAND health insurance experiment found that adults who used more medical services because their insurance plan did not require copayments did not have statistically significant better health status than adults in health plans with lower use rates (Brook et al. 1983).

Indemnity insurance also places an annual limit (referred to as a "stop loss"), for example, $1,500, on the patient's responsibility for out-of-pocket payments. If a patient has a serious illness, that out-of-pocket maximum is reached fairly early in the treatment process. After that point, both the patient and their physician (assuming fee-for-service payment) have an incentive to try all types of treatments that may provide some benefit to the patient, no matter how small that benefit. The expression "flat-of-the-curve medicine" came to indicate the use of all medical technology even though the benefit derived by the patient was extremely small. The only cost to the patient is nonfinancial, the discomfort and risk associated with the treatment. It is not surprising, therefore, that medical expenditures for those who are seriously ill are extraordinarily high. Patients in such circumstances have everything available to them that modern medicine can provide.

The problem of moral hazard has plagued health insurers. It has resulted in excessive use, increased the cost of medical care, and raised insurance premiums. Until the 1980s, the primary method used by health insurers to control moral hazard was to require the patient to pay a deductible and part of the cost themselves, by use of a copayment. During the 1980s insurers began to use more aggressive methods to control "overuse" of medical services, such as prior authorization before a patient could be admitted to the hospital, utilization review once the patient was hospitalized, and second surgical opinions. Unless prior authorization was received, the patient would be liable for part of the hospitalization cost (and often the patient's physician had to spend time justifying the procedure to the insurer). Second surgical opinions were an attempt to provide the patient and the insurer with more information as to the value of the recommended surgical procedure.

These cost-containment or rationing techniques are often referred to as "managed care." More recent managed care methods include case management, which minimizes the medical cost of catastrophic medical cases, and preferred physician panels, which exclude physicians who overuse medical services. These provider panels are then marketed to employer groups as being less costly, thereby offering subscribers lower insurance premiums if they restrict their choice of physician to members of the panel.

In addition to changing patient incentives and relying on managed care techniques, moral hazard can also be controlled by changing physicians' incentives. Health maintenance organizations (HMOs) are paid an annual fee for providing medical services to their enrolled population. The out-of-pocket price to the enrollee for use of services in an HMO is very low; consequently usage rates would be expected to be very high. Since the HMO bears the risk that their enrollees' medical services will not exceed their annual payment, the HMO has an incentive not to provide "excessive" amounts of medical services. The HMO patient must instead be concerned with receiving too little care. HMO physicians ration care based on the physician's perception of the benefits to the patient and the full costs to the HMO of further treatment. Since HMO enrollees have very low copayments, the onus (and incentives) for decreasing moral hazard, hence rationing care, is placed on the HMO's physicians.

These insurance company and HMO approaches to decreasing moral hazard attempt to match the additional benefit of medical services to their full cost. Copayments and financial penalties for not receiving prior authorization are incentives to change the patient's behavior. In an HMO, the HMO's physicians are responsible for controlling moral hazard.

Differences between Rationing Methods

There are important differences between government rationing of services and the rationing (by price) that occurs in the private market. In a private system, patients differ on the value they place on additional medical services; however, those who place a higher value on those services can always purchase more services. As their incomes increase, they may prefer to spend more of their additional income on medical care than on other goods and services. If an HMO is too slow to adopt new technology or too stringent on access to medical services provided to its enrollees, those enrollees can switch to another HMO or to indemnity insurance, pay higher premiums, and receive more services.

Under a system of government rationing, if a patient places a higher value than does the government on additional medical services and the patient is willing to pay the full cost of those services, the patient will still be unable to purchase them.

Medical services must be rationed, since society cannot afford to provide all the medical services that would be demanded at zero price. Which rationing mechanism should be used: by having people pay for additional services and by voluntarily joining an HMO or a managed care organization, or, alternatively, by the government deciding on the availability of medical resources? The first, or market approach, permits subscribers to match their costs to the value they place on additional services. It is only when the government decides on the costs and benefits of medical services that availability will be lower than desired by those who value medical services more highly, and those persons are not permitted the choice of spending more of their own resources on medical services. Choice of rationing technique, relying on the private sector versus the government, is essential for determining how much medical care will be provided, to whom, and at what cost.

Regardless of which rationing approach is used for allocating re- sources to medical care, a knowledge of price sensitivity is important for public policy and for attaining efficiency. If the government wants to in- crease the use of preventive services such as prenatal care, mammograms, and dental checkups, for underserved populations, would lowering the price (and waiting cost) of such services achieve that goal? Would raising the out-of-pocket price for some visits by insurers decrease the use of care that is of low value? And if it were desired to stimulate competition among health plans, how much of a difference in their premiums would cause large numbers of employees to switch plans? If consumers are to be able to match the benefits and costs from use of medical services, they must not only have information on each health plan, but they must also be faced with the costs of their decisions; they will then be more discriminating in their choice of health plan and in use of services.

References

Aaron, H., and W. B. Schwartz. "Rationing Health Care: The Choice before Us." *Science* 247 (26 January 1990): 418–22.
Brook, R. H., J. Ware, W. H. Rogers, E. B. Keeler, A. R. Davies, C. A. Donald, G. A. Goldberg, K. N. Lohr, P. C. Masthay, and J. P. Newhouse. "Does Free Care Improve Adults' Health? Results from a Randomized Controlled Trial." *The New England Journal of Medicine* 309 (December 1983): 1426–34.
Long, S. H., R. F. Settle, and C. W. Wrightson. "Employee Premiums, Availability of Alternative Plans, and HMO Disenrollment," *Medical Care* 26 (October 1988): 927–38.

6

How Much Health Insurance
Should Everyone Have?

Why do some people have health insurance that covers almost all their medical expenditures, including dental and vision care, while others do not? Why does the government subsidize the purchase of private health insurance for those with high incomes? Has health insurance stimulated the growth in medical expenditures, or has it merely served as protection against rapidly rising medical expenses? The answers to these questions are important for explaining the rapid increase in medical expenditures, as well as for understanding proposals for health care reform.

The purpose of health insurance is to enable people to get rid of uncertainty, the possibility that they would incur a large medical expense. They are able to convert this possibility of a large loss into a certain, but small, loss by buying health insurance. Insurance spreads risk among a large number of people and when each person pays a premium, the aggregate amount of the premiums are able to cover the large losses of relatively few people.

Definitions of Insurance Terms

Before going on, it is useful to define a number of terms. *Indemnity insurance* reimburses either the health provider or the patient a fixed amount (or a percentage of the bill) when the insured patient receives a medical treatment. When the insured patient has a *service benefit* policy, the insurer pays the provider for the services needed by the patient.

Health insurance policies today typically contain both indemnity and service benefit features. Physician services and out-of-hospital services are usually treated as indemnity insurance, while hospital admissions are usually paid for as a service benefit.

The difference between the provider's charge and the insurance payment is for deductibles and copayments. A *deductible* is a given dollar amount of money that the patient will have to spend before the insurer will pay any medical expenses. Typically, indemnity policies require that an insured family spend between $250 and $500 of their own money before the insurer will start paying part of their medical bills. A deductible lowers the insurance premium because it eliminates the many small medical expenses that most families have each year. The insurer is also able to lower its administrative costs by eliminating the claims processing for handling a large number of small claims.

The effect of a deductible on the insurance premium is illustrated in Figure 6.1. On the vertical axis are the percent of families having a medical expense. On the horizontal axis is the size of a medical expense incurred in any year. Thus a large percent of families have relatively small medical expenses, while a small percent of families have a very large (referred to as *catastrophic*) expense. Eliminating the area designated as a deductible would reduce the overall amount spent on medical care, thereby reducing the insurance premium.

Ideally (although it is not often done), a deductible should be related to a family's income, for example, 1 percent of their annual income. A

Figure 6.1   Deductibles, Copayments, and Catastrophic Expenses

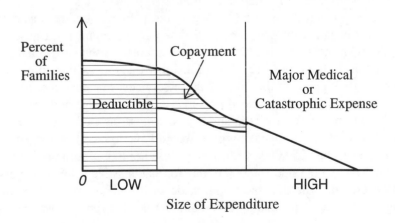

deductible that is the same for everyone could turn out to be a financial hardship to low-income families but not for high-income families, who could afford to have a larger deductible.

When a patient pays a percentage of the physician's bill, for example, 20 percent, then this is referred to as *cost sharing* or a *copayment*. Copayments provide the patient with an incentive to be sensitive to physicians' charges, perhaps by shopping around, since the patient will have to pay part of the bill. The patient will also have an incentive to use fewer services because he or she will have to balance the value of an additional visit against its cost (copayment). Copayments also reduce the insurer's share of medical expenses, as shown in Figure 6.1. Indemnity policies are typically 80/20 plans, meaning that the insurer pays 80 percent of the bill and the patient pays 20 percent. Indemnity policies also contain a *stop loss*, which places an overall limit on the patient's out-of-pocket expenses. For example, once a patient has paid a deductible and copayments that add up to, for example, $2,000, the insurer pays 100 percent of all remaining expenses during that year. Without a stop loss, unlimited copayments could become a financial hardship. Copayments typically apply to use of out-of-hospital services considered to be discretionary.

Catastrophic claims comprise the tail of medical expenditures, as shown in Figure 6.1, that are incurred by only a small percent of families. The definition of a catastrophic expense depends on the patient's family income, since a $2,000 expense may be a catastrophic expense to some families but not others. Ideally, the definition of a catastrophic expense should also be related to family income, but few policies do so. Insurance policies that cover only catastrophic medical expenses may be thought of as policies with very high deductibles.

The amount of medical expenditures paid out by the insurance company is called the *pure premium*. The pure premium for a group of people with the same risk level (age/sex) represents their expected cost of a medical expense, which is the probability that they will need medical services multiplied by the cost of those services. For example, assume that the probability of my needing surgery (given my age and sex) were 5 percent and the cost of the surgery, if it were needed, was $50,000, then I (and others in my risk group) would have to pay a pure premium of $2,500 a year ($50,000 × .05). If I chose not to buy insurance, then I would have to put aside $50,000 to pay for that possible medical expense. However, I may not be able to put aside such a large amount—or even larger amounts as, for example, the amount needed for a transplant—or

I may not want to tie up my funds in that way. Insurance offers me an alternative; it permits me to pay a premium that is equivalent to budgeting for an uncertain medical expense. I can eliminate the uncertainty of a large medical expense by paying an annual premium.

When everyone in a particular group has the same chance of becoming ill and incurring a medical expense, each person is considered to be in the same risk class and would be charged the same pure premium. The *actual premium* charged, however, is always greater than the pure premium because the insurer has to recover its administrative and marketing costs, as well as earn a profit. This difference between the pure and actual premium is referred to as the *loading charge*.

Insurance-Purchasing Decision Making

The size of the loading charge oftens determines why people buy insurance for some medical expenses but not for others. If people could buy insurance at the pure premium, we would buy insurance for almost everything, since it would reflect, on average, what they would likely spend anyway. However, when I am charged more than the pure premium, I have to decide whether I want to buy insurance or to self-insure, that is, bear the risk myself. The higher the loading charge, relative to the pure premium, the less insurance I would buy. For example, part of the loading charge is related to the administrative cost of processing a claim, which is not too different for a small or a large claim. Small claims, therefore, have larger loading costs (relative to their pure premium) than do large claims. People are more willing to pay a large administrative cost for a large than a small claim.

In the above example where the pure premium was $2,500 a year, even if the insurance company charged me $2,600 a year ($100 above the pure premium), I would probably buy the insurance than bear the risk myself. However, my decision would be different with a smaller expected medical expense. I would rather put aside $200 a year for my family's dental visits than pay the same $100 administrative cost, which would be equal to 50 percent of the pure premium ($200 pure premium plus a $100 loading charge would equal a premium of $300). In this second case I would rather bear the risk myself than buy insurance.

The above discussion suggests that people are likely to buy insurance for large, unexpected medical expenses, rather than for small medical expenses (for a more complete discussion of the factors affecting the demand for health insurance, see Feldstein 1993). This is the pattern typically observed in the purchase of health insurance. A hospital admission and physician expenses connected with that hospital admission, such as the surgeon's and anesthesiologist's fees, are more completely covered by insurance than are expenses for a physician's office visit. Thus an important characteristic of good insurance is that it cover large catastrophic expenses. A person is less able to afford the catastrophic costs of a major illness or accident than front-end or first-dollar coverage, which are typically small expenses with relatively high loading charges.

Tax-Free Employer-Paid Insurance

Surprisingly, however, we also observe that many people have insurance against small claims, such as dental visits, physician office visits, and vision services. How can we explain this?

Advantages

The predominant source of health insurance coverage for those less than 65 years is through the workplace, where 85 percent of all private health insurance is purchased by the employer on behalf of the employee. The reason for this is that the federal tax code does not consider employer-paid health insurance to be part of the employee's taxable income; it is exempt from federal, state, and Social Security taxes.

Until the early 1980s, marginal tax rates for federal income taxes were as high as 70 percent. Throughout the late 1960s and 1970s inflation was increasing and pushing employees into higher marginal tax brackets. Social Security taxes have also been steadily rising; currently, the employer and employee each pay 7.65 percent of the employee's wage, up to a maximum wage of $57,600. Employees as well as the employer had a financial incentive for additional compensation to be provided in the form of health insurance benefits rather than cash income. The employer saved their share of Social Security taxes while employees did not have to pay federal, state, or Social Security taxes on additional health insurance benefits.

For example, assume an employee was in a 30 percent tax bracket, had to pay 5 percent state income tax, and 7 percent Social Security tax, already had basic hospital and medical coverage, and was due to receive a $1,000 raise. That employee would be left with only $580 after taxes to purchase dental care and other medical services not covered by insurance for his or her family. However, if the employer used that $1,000 to purchase additional health insurance to cover these same out-of-pocket payments instead of raising the employee's income, the employee could use the complete $1,000 to buy those services that he or she would have had to purchase with after-tax dollars. The employee would be able to pay the $580 with before-tax income and still have several hundred dollars available to cover additional out-of-pocket medical expenses.

Higher-income employees had even greater incentives to substitute more comprehensive insurance coverage for wage increases. Imagine someone in a 50 percent tax bracket (before 1980) with the same state and Social Security taxes. A $1,000 raise would leave them with only $380 to purchase dental, vision, and mental health services, whereas the full $1,000 could be spent on those services if it were used to buy additional health insurance.

As employees moved into higher tax brackets, the higher loading charge on small claims was more than offset by using before-tax income to buy health insurance for those small claims. Using the earlier example of dental care, the choice was between spending $200 of after-tax income on dental care or buying dental insurance for $300. Spending $200 on my family's dental care would require me to earn $350 in before-tax income (30 percent federal tax, 5 percent state, and 7 percent Social Security tax). However, if my employer used that same $350 and purchased dental benefits for me, it would more than cover the premium, including the $200 loading charge, and leave $50 to buy even more medical services. Tax-free employer-purchased health insurance provided a financial incentive to purchase health insurance for small claims.

Another way of viewing the tax subsidy for health insurance is as follows: If an employee saves 40 percent when the employer buys health insurance, then the price of insurance to that employee has been reduced by 40 percent. Studies indicate that the purchase of insurance has an approximate proportional relationship to changes in its price (Pauly 1986). Thus a 40 percent price reduction would be expected to increase the quantity of insurance purchased by 40 percent.

The advantages of tax-free employer-purchased health insurance stimulated the demand for comprehensive health insurance coverage, particularly among higher-income employees. In some high-income employee groups, such as the United Automobile Workers (UAW), deductibles and copayments became smaller and disappeared. More services, not traditionally thought of as insurable, such as for small routine expenditures, became part of the employee's health insurance.

Consequences

There were important consequences to the greater comprehensiveness of employer-purchased health insurance. First, "too many" services were covered by health insurance. Administrative costs increased as the insurer had to process many small claims that would have been excluded by a deductible. To process a $20 prescription drug claim cost the same as a much larger medical expense. Second, as insurance became more comprehensive, the patient's concern with the prices charged for medical services decreased. Physicians, hospitals, and other health providers could more easily raise their charges, since "it was covered by insurance"— someone else was paying for it. Similarly, as the amount they had to pay out-of-pocket for their medical expenses declined, patients increased their use of those services, sought more referrals to specialists, and underwent extensive medical testing.

The growth of health insurance and medical technology was intertwined. Expensive technology, which increases the cost of a medical expense, causes people to buy health insurance to protect themselves from those large unexpected medical expenses. At the same time, the availability of insurance to pay for expensive technology stimulated its development. When comprehensive insurance removes any concern the insured person may have with the cost of their care, they (and their physician acting on their behalf) want access to the latest technology, as long as it offers some additional benefit, no matter how small. The benefits of that technology to the patient outweighed their out-of-pocket costs of using it. Because insurance was available to pay the costs of expensive technology, such as transplants, there were financial incentives to develop benefit-producing technology. Thus medical technology was stimulated by, and in turn stimulated, the purchase of health insurance.

Conversely, until recently, there was little interest in cost-reducing technology because employers could pass higher insurance costs on to employees, in the form of reduced wages, or in higher prices to consumers. Also, the after-tax value of savings to employees from undertaking stringent cost-containment measures was small. If, for example, insurance premiums could be reduced by $300 by limiting employees' choice of physician, the after-tax savings of $150 was probably not worth the inconvenience to the employee and his or her family associated with changing physicians.

The lack of concern over the price of medical services and the increased use of those services caused medical expenditures to sharply increase, which, in turn, caused health insurance premiums to rapidly rise. Higher insurance premiums meant smaller wage increases, but this was not obvious to employees, since the employer was paying the insurance premium.

Hundreds of billions of dollars of tax revenues have been lost because of employer-paid health insurance. Currently, the federal government loses $45 billion in tax revenues and $27 billion in lost Social Security taxes a year because employer-paid health insurance is not considered part of the employee's taxable income. These lost tax revenues primarily benefit high-income employees since they are in higher tax brackets. As shown in Table 6.1, the higher the employee's income, the greater is the value of the exclusion from income of employer-purchased health insurance. This $72 billion in lost tax revenues is equivalent to a huge federal subsidy for the purchase of health insurance to those who can most easily afford it. In contrast, the federal government spends $80 billion on Medicaid, which is a means-tested program for the poor.

Finally, tax-free employer-paid health insurance reduced employees' incentive to choose lower-cost health plans. Many employers paid the entire premium of any plan selected by the employee (or the employer contributed more than the premium of the lowest-cost plan offered) and since there was no visible cost to the employee, the employee's incentive was to choose the most comprehensive plan with easiest access to

Table 6.1   Value of Health Care Exclusion for Typical Families, 1991

Family Income	Valued Tax Exclusion
less than $10,000	$ 50
$10,000–$14,999	207
$15,000–$19,999	366
$20,000–$29,999	594
$30,000–$39,999	857
$40,000–$49,999	986
$50,000–$74,999	1,373
$75,000–$99,999	1,427
$100,000 or more	1,463
All families	$ 802

Reprinted with permission of Lewin/VHI (Fairfax, VA); unpublished estimates using the Health Benefits Simulation Model.

physicians and specialists. Health plans have not had financial incentives to compete on premiums.

Proposed Limitation of Tax-Free Status

To encourage competition among health plans on the basis of access to services, quality, and premiums, employees have to pay out-of-pocket the additional cost of a more expensive health plan. The employee will then evaluate whether the additional benefits of that plan are worth its additional costs. Unless a limit is placed on the amount of the employer's contribution that is considered to be tax free, many employees will continue to select health plans based on their benefits without regard to their premiums. Competition among health plans based on premiums, reputation, and access to services will not occur until the employee has a greater financial stake in their decision.

It is not surprising that economists favor eliminating, or at least limiting, the tax-exempt status of employer-paid health insurance. No longer would those with higher incomes receive a subsidy for their purchase of health insurance. Instead, increased tax revenues would come from those who have benefited most, namely those with higher incomes. These funds could then be used to subsidize health insurance for those with low incomes. Employees, using after-tax dollars, would make more cost-conscious choices in their use of services and in their choice of health plans.

One likely outcome of increased price sensitivity by employees (or employers acting on their behalf) is that health insurance coverage would become less comprehensive. It would no longer be worthwhile to buy insurance for small claims that have relatively large loading charges. Consequently, dental and vision services would likely be dropped from insurance policies. Deductibles will be increased on out-of-hospital services, thereby decreasing administrative costs and insurance premiums. Copayments will also be common, both as a means of decreasing the insurance premium and for controlling use of services. Those employees who prefer to have comprehensive benefits and not pay large copayments will be more likely to join capitated systems, such as HMOs, where the decision on use of services is made by the provider, rather than by the patient.

Whether patients become more price sensitive because of copayments or they delegate the decision to restrict use of services to their HMO, use of services will decline. The basis for making treatment decisions will change. No longer will use of services and choice of health plan be based only on a consideration of their benefits. Employees (and physicians in HMOs) will also have to consider the costs of their choices.

References

Feldstein, P. J. *Health Care Economics,* 4th ed. Albany, New York: Delmar Publishers Inc., 1993.
Pauly, M.V. "Taxation, Health Insurance, and Market Failure in the Medical Economy." *Journal of Economic Literature* 24 (June 1986): 644.

7

Why Are Those Who Most
Need Health Insurance
Least Able to Buy It?

We have all heard stories of individuals who are sick and need, for example, open-heart surgery, but no insurance company will sell them health insurance. Health insurance seems to be available only for those who do not need it. Should health insurance companies be required to sell insurance to those who are sick and need it most?

To understand these issues, as well as what would be appropriate public policy, it is necessary to understand how insurance premiums are determined and how health insurance markets work.

Determining Insurance Premiums

Most private health insurance (85 percent) is purchased through the workplace. The insurance premium paid by an employer on behalf of its employees consists of (1) the loading charge, which represents approximately 8 percent of the premium, and (2) the claims experience of the employee group, which comprises the remaining 92 percent of the premium (see Figure 7.1). The loading charge reflects the insurance company's marketing costs, administrative costs of handling the insurance claims, and profit for the insurance company. The claims experience of an employee group is the number of claims submitted by members of that group multiplied by the average cost per claim. The claims experience

Figure 7.1   The Determinants of Health Insurance Premiums

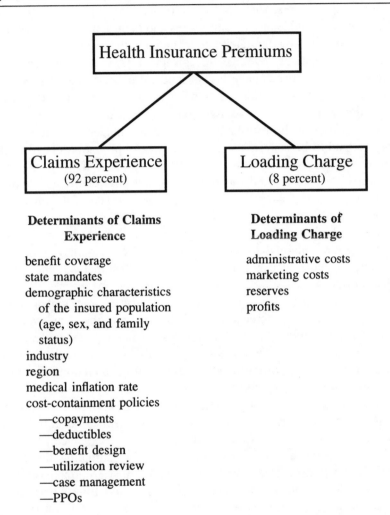

portion of the premium is the total medical expenditures paid out by the insurer on behalf of the group. Differences in premiums among employee groups, as well as the annual rise in employer health insurance premiums, result primarily from differences in claims experience. When the premium is based on the claims experience of the particular group, the premium is *experience rated*.

When a new group applies for health insurance, the insurer attempts to estimate the likely claims experience of the group. As shown in Figure 7.1, the insurer will consider factors that affect the group's medical expenditures, such as the following: the types of medical and other benefits provided to the employees and their dependents; the type of mandates required by the state to be included in the insurance policy, such as hair transplants or coverage for chiropractors; the average age of the group (older employees have higher medical expenditures than younger employees); the proportion of females (females have higher medical expenditures than males at younger ages and less at older age levels); the industry in which the firm competes (doctors, nurses, accountants, and lawyers tend to be heavier users of health care, probably related to their educational levels, than bank tellers); the region of the country where the employees are located (hospital costs and physician fees are higher on the West Coast than in the South); and an estimate of the growth rate in medical inflation.

Once an insurer has insured a group long enough to have a history of that group's claims experience, the insurance company will project that claims experience and multiply it by an estimate of the medical inflation rate.

Various approaches can be used to reduce a group's claims experience. For example, increasing the deductible and the coinsurance rate will decrease employees' use of services; expanding insurance benefits to include lower-cost substitutes to inpatient admissions will lower treatment costs; and requiring utilization review of hospital admissions, case management of catastrophic cases, and use of PPO providers will lower use rates and provider charges. Thus, the claims experience of a group is related to the characteristics of that group, the medical benefits covered, and the cost-containment methods included in the insurance policy.

The insurer bears the risk of incorrectly estimating the group's medical experience. If the premium charged to that group is too low, the insurer will lose money. Insurance companies and Blue Cross have in the past lost a great deal of money by underestimating claims experience and the medical inflation rate. An insurer cannot merely increase the premiums of the group in the following period to recover their losses because the insurance market is price competitive. If an insurer says to an employer, "We need to increase our profit this coming year because we lost money on your employees last year," the employer may switch to a competitor or to an HMO.

Even if the claims experience of two employee groups is similar, one group may have a lower insurance premium because it has a lower loading charge. Larger groups have smaller loading charges because administrative and marketing costs, which are generally fixed, are spread over a larger number of employees. Also, insurers earn a lower profit when they insure larger groups because they fear that if their profit is too high, large groups will decide to self-insure by bearing the risk themselves. Smaller groups, on the other hand, are less likely to be able to bear the risk of self-insurance. If a very large claim were to occur in one year, the financial burden may be too large for a small group to bear. In a larger group, large claims are likely to be offset by premiums from employees making only small or no claims in a given year. In addition to being able to charge small groups a higher profit, an insurer is likely to maintain a higher reserve in case there is a large claim, thereby further increasing the loading charge for small groups. However, the amount of profit the insurer is able to charge small groups is limited by competition from other insurers and health maintenance organizations (HMOs).

How Health Insurance Markets Work

With this brief description of how insurance premiums are determined, we can examine why those who are ill find it difficult to buy insurance.

Adverse Selection

Let us assume that an individual without health insurance requires a heart transplant and tries to purchase health insurance. If the insurer does not know that the person requires expensive medical treatment, the person's premium will be based on the claims experience of persons in a similar age (risk) group. This difference in information between the individual and the insurer about the individual's health status can lead to *adverse selection*, that is, a person in ill health will attempt to conceal that information from the insurer so that the insurer will not know their true risk.

For example, if there were 100 people in a risk group, each with a 1 percent chance of needing a medical treatment whose cost would be $100,000, then the premium for each (without the loading charge) would be $1,000 (.01 × $100,000). Each year one member of the group would require a $100,000 treatment. Now if a person who needs that particular treatment (whose risk is 100 percent) is permitted to join that group at a premium of $1,000 (based on a mistaken risk level of .01), the person with the high risk receives a subsidy of $99,000, since their premium, based on their risk level, should have been $100,000. Since the $1,000 premium was based on a risk level of 1 percent, the insurer collected insufficient premiums to pay for the second $100,000 expense. The insurer loses $99,000.

This example does not differ from one in which a man learns that he has a terminal illness and, unbeknownst to the insurer, decides to purchase a $1,000,000 life insurance policy to provide for his wife and children. Or a person whose home has burnt down decides to buy fire insurance. Insurance enables a person to insure against uncertainty. But once uncertainty no longer exists, the person's need for a heart transplant is not insurable.

If the insurance company knew that the individual wanted health insurance to cover the costs of a heart transplant, then the insurance company would charge a premium that reflected the person's expected claims experience, that is, the individual's premium would be equal to the cost of the heart transplant plus a loading charge.

We all favor subsidizing those who cannot afford, but need, an expensive treatment. Similarly, we favor subsidies to poor families. However, is it not more appropriate for the government, rather than the insurer, to provide those subsidies? When insurers are made to bear such losses, they will eventually be forced out of business unless they can protect themselves from persons who withhold information and claim to be in lower-risk groups.

To protect themselves against adverse selection (insuring high-risk persons for premiums mistakenly based on those with low risks), the insurer could raise everyone's premium, but then many low-risk subscribers, who would be willing to pay $1,000 but not $2,000 for a 1 percent risk, would drop their insurance. As more low-risk subscribers drop out, premiums for remaining subscribers will increase further, causing still more low-risk subscribers to drop out. Eventually large numbers of low-risk persons would be uninsured, even though they would be willing to pay an actuarially fair premium, based on their (low) risk group.

Instead, an insurer may attempt to learn as much as the patient about the patient's health status. Examining and testing the individual who wants to buy health insurance is a means of equalizing the information between the two parties. Another means insurers use to protect themselves against adverse selection, that is, from misclassifying high risks into low-risk groups, is by stating that their insurance coverage will not apply to *preexisting conditions*, which are medical conditions known by the patient to exist and to require medical treatment. Similarly, an insurer might use a delay of benefits clause or waiting period; for example, obstetrical benefits may not be covered until a policy has been in effect 10 months. Large deductibles will also discourage high-risk individuals since they will realize that they have to pay a large amount of their expenses themselves.

Insurers are less concerned about adverse selection when selling insurance to large groups with low employee turnover. In such groups, health insurance is provided by the employer and is a tax-free benefit (subsidized by the government); the total group includes all the low risks as well. Typically, individuals join large companies more for other attributes of the job than for health insurance coverage. And once in the employer group, employees cannot just drop the group insurance when well and buy it when ill. Thus, for insurance companies, adverse selection is more of a concern when individuals or very small groups (with typically higher turnover) want to buy insurance. For example, an insurer might be concerned that the owner of a small firm might hire family members who become ill so as to receive insurance benefits. Thus employees with preexisting medical conditions will be denied coverage because insurers will use testing and exclusions to protect themselves against adverse selection.

Some state and local governments have attempted to assist individuals with preexisting conditions by prohibiting insurers from using tests to determine, for example, whether an individual is HIV positive. Rather than subsidizing care for such individuals themselves, these governments have tried to shift the medical costs to the insurer and their other subscribers. This is an inequitable way of subsidizing care for those with preexisting conditions since many insured, but low-risk, subscribers have low incomes. It would be fairer if the government used an income-related tax to provide the subsidy. Another consequence of government regulations that shift the cost of those who are ill to insurers and their subscribers is that insurers will rely on other types of restrictions, not covered by the regulations, to protect themselves, such as delay of benefits and exclusion of certain occupations, industries, or geographic areas.

There are several reasons why individuals, even though they are healthy, do not have health insurance. An insurance premium that is much higher than the expected claims experience of an individual will make that insurance too expensive. For example, if an employee is not part of a large insured group, they will be charged a higher insurance premium because they are suspected by the insurer of being a high risk. Also, the loading charge will be higher for the self-employed and those in small groups because the insurer's administration and marketing costs are spread over fewer employees, leading to a higher premium. Further, state insurance mandates that require expensive benefits or more practitioners be included in all insurance sold in that state result in higher insurance premiums; consequently fewer people are willing to buy such insurance. Many individuals and members of small groups also lack insurance coverage because premiums are too high relative to their incomes. Such persons would rather rely on Medicaid if they become ill. Then there are those who can afford to purchase insurance but choose not to; if they become ill, they become a burden on the taxpayer.

The best way to eliminate the problem of adverse selection is to require everyone to have health insurance. Subsidies to purchase insurance can be provided to those with low incomes and to those who are high risk in relation to their income. Under mandatory health insurance, most individuals would be good risks when they purchased health insurance and would not wait until they were ill and hence uninsurable. Everyone would have health insurance when they needed it, and when insurance companies did impose delay of benefit restrictions on new enrollees, enrollees with preexisting conditions would remain with their current insurer until their medical condition had been taken care of.

Preferred-Risk Selection

Just as insurers want to protect themselves against bad risks, they also clearly prefer insuring individuals who are better-than-average risks. As long as different groups and individuals pay the *same* premium, even though their risks vary, insurers have an incentive to seek out those who have lower than average risks. This is referred to as *preferred-risk selection.*

As shown in Table 7.1, 1 percent of the population incurs 30 percent of total health expenditures. (Fifty percent of those in the top 1 percent are over the age of 65.) In 1963 1 percent of the population incurred only 17 percent of total expenditures, which indicates the effect that medical technology has on increasing medical expenditures. Five percent of the population incurs 58 percent of total expenditures. Given this high concentration of expenditures among a small percent of the population, an insurer could greatly increase their profits, as well as avoid losses, by trying to avoid the most costly patients. An insurer able to select enrollees among the 50 percent of the population that incurs only 3 percent of total expenditures will greatly profit. The only way to provide insurers with an incentive to take the high-risk, hence costly, patients is to provide insurers with *risk-adjusted premiums*. Insurers would then have an incentive to try and minimize the cost of treating these patients, rather than searching for low-risk enrollees.

There are several ways in which insurers attempt to enroll better-than-average risks when the premium is the same for all risks. For example, if everyone enrolling in a particular HMO pays the same annual premium, then the HMO would prefer those groups who have lower-than-average claims experience, who are in low-risk industries, and who are younger-than-average employees. To encourage younger subscribers, the HMO might emphasize services used by younger couples, such as prenatal and well-baby care. Emphasizing wellness and sports medicine programs is also likely to draw a healthier population. Similarly, deem-phasizing its tertiary care facilities for heart disease and cancer treatment sends a message to those who are older and at higher risk for those illnesses. Further, locating its clinics and physicians in areas where lower-risk populations reside also results in a biased (favorable) selection of subscribers.

Those on Medicare can voluntarily decide to join an HMO; if they decide to change their mind, they can leave the HMO with only one month's notice. When an HMO determines that a Medicare patient requires high-cost treatment, it may encourage the patient to disenroll

Table 7.1 Distribution of Health Expenditures for the U.S. Population by Magnitude of Expenditures, Selected Years, 1928–1987

Percent of U.S. Population Ranked by Expenditures	*1928*	*1963*	*1970*	*1977*	*1980*	*1987*
Top 1 percent	—	17%	26%	27%	29%	30%
Top 2 percent	—	—	35	38	39	41
Top 5 percent	52	43	50	55	55	58
Top 10 percent	—	59	66	70	70	72
Top 30 percent	93	—	88	90	90	91
Top 50 percent	—	95	96	97	96	97
Bottom 50 percent	—	5	4	3	4	3

This table is reprinted with the publisher's permission: *Health Affairs*, 7500 Old Georgetown Road, Suite 600, Bethesda, MD 20814, 301-656-7401. See Winter 1992 issue, "The Concentration of Health Expenditures: An Update" by M. L. Berk and A. C. Monheit.

by suggesting that he or she might possibly benefit from more suitable treatment for the condition outside the HMO. By eliminating these high-cost subscribers, an HMO could save a great deal of money. To discourage some HMOs from using this approach to maintain only the most favorable Medicare risks, the one-month notice should be repealed or the HMO should be held responsible for reimbursing the non-HMO providers when Medicare patients disenroll.

Improving the Health Insurance Market

Biased selection, both adverse and preferred-risk selection, are problems in the health insurance market. They occur because of differences in information on health status, consumer choice of health plans, and fixed premiums for subscribers whose expected medical expenses differ from the average cost per subscriber.

Several proposals have been made for improving the health insurance market.[1] One is to require all insurers "community rate" their subscribers, that is, charge all their subscribers the same premium regardless of health status or other risk factors. The cost of higher-risk individuals would be spread among all subscribers. Community rating, however, provides insurers with even stronger incentives to select preferred risks. Further, with uniform premiums, regardless of risk status, insurers and employers would no longer have an incentive to encourage risk-reducing behavior among their subscribers and employees, such as providing smoking cessation and wellness programs; premiums for employee groups could not be reduced relative to other groups who do not invest in such cost-reducing behavior. Sky divers, motorcyclists, and others who engage in risky behavior are subsidized by those who attempt to lower their risks. Rather than reducing the cost of risky behavior, higher premiums for those who engage in higher-risk activities would provide them with an incentive to reduce such behavior and to bear the full cost of their activities.

Community rating also has serious equity effects. A community-rated system benefits those who are at high risk and penalizes those who are at low risk. Those at lower risk pay higher premiums, while those at higher risk pay lower premiums, than under an experience-rated system. Those at higher risk are subsidized, in effect, by placing a tax on those who are lower risk. Since these "subsidies and taxes" are based on risk rather than income, low-risk individuals who also have low incomes will end up subsidizing some higher-risk, higher-income people. Not all high risks are poor, and not all low risks are wealthy.

A second proposal to improve the health insurance market is to require insurers to offer *guaranteed renewability* within standard "rate bands," that is, upon renewal, premium increases can vary from the average increase in premiums by only plus or minus 20 percent. These proposals would make insurers sell "real" insurance. A person buys insurance to decrease uncertainty. If they become ill and the insurer does not renew their insurance or charges them a very high premium, their initial purchase of insurance has not decreased their uncertainty. Unless they are able to renew their insurance, they will not be protected from a large unexpected loss.

Summary

Adverse and preferred-risk selection occur because the individual's risk is not reflected in their premium. These selection problems would be minimized if premiums were related to risk levels. Then insurers would not need to reject high risks or to search for low risks. (And, in the case of adverse selection, the problem would be eliminated if everyone were required to have health insurance.) Government regulations, such as the elimination of testing and mandating community rating for insurers, have indirect effects that may worsen equity, decrease risk-reducing behavior by employers, and lead to offsetting actions by insurers.

Adverse and preferred-risk selection affect subscribers and health insurers. To solve these problems, one must be aware of why biased selection occurs. Proposed solutions should be evaluated on the basis of whether they encourage risk-reducing behavior, include incentives for efficient utilization of medical services, and impose a burden on those with low incomes, who may also be low risk. Lastly, health insurance reform should be directed toward eliminating uncertainty, which is what people want when they buy health insurance.

Note

1. These proposals are directed toward improving the health insurance market for small employee groups and assume that these small groups can afford to purchase health insurance. Financing health care for the poor is discussed in later chapters, as are other aspects of health care reform, such as competitive medical systems and malpractice.

8

Medicare and Medicaid

In 1965 Congress enacted two different financing programs to cover two separate population groups, the aged and the poor. As a result, the federal government's role in the financing of personal medical services increased dramatically. Prior to the introduction of Medicare (acute hospital and medical care for the aged) and Medicaid (medical services for the poor), the states were responsible for medical services to the indigent while the federal government supported the VA hospital system and medical services for federal employees and their dependents.

Medicare and Medicaid increased the government's role in health care, increasing government expenditures (both state and federal) from 20 percent to 40 percent of total medical expenditures. In 1992 the federal government spent $223 billion for medical services, compared to $3.6 billion in 1965. The increasing role of the federal government (accounting for three-fourths of total, federal and state, government health expenditures) and the rapid annual percent increase in government medical expenditures (15 percent in 1992) are the reasons for the federal government's attempts to reduce the rise in medical expenditures.

The Current State of Medicaid

Medicaid is a welfare program for the poor. It is administered by each state, but the federal government pays between 50 percent and 80 percent matching funds (on average 57 percent), based on each state's per capita income. To qualify for federal matching funds, each state must cover certain federally mandated population groups, such as single-parent families eligible for Aid to Families with Dependent Children (AFDC), low-income pregnant women and children, and low-income aged, blind, and disabled persons who qualify for Supplemental Security Income. In recent years Congress has broadened the eligible population groups, such as including pregnant women and infants with incomes up to 185 percent of the federal poverty level. These broadened eligibility requirements have caused the number of eligibles to increase from 22 million in 1988 to 27 million in 1991. In addition, in recent years high-cost patients, such as AIDS sufferers and crack babies, have caused state and federal Medicaid expenditures to sharply increase, from $51.6 billion in 1988 to $120 billion in 1992.

Although more than 70 percent of Medicaid recipients are low-income parents and children, they account for only 29 percent of Medicaid expenditures. The remaining 70 percent of Medicaid expenditures are for institutional care for the aged, disabled, and mentally retarded (see Figure 8.1).

Figure 8.1   Percent Distribution of Medicaid Recipients and Medicaid Vendor Payments by Eligibility Status, 1991

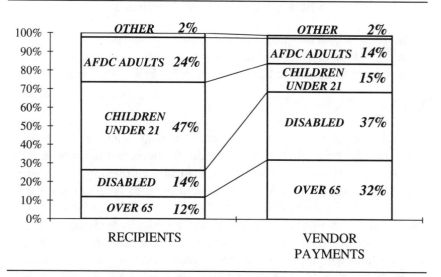

Source: U.S. Department of Health and Human Services, Health Care Financing Administration (Washington, DC), *Medicaid Statistics, Fiscal Year 1991.*

Medicaid is generally perceived as being inadequate. Only those with very low incomes are eligible; no more than 42 percent of people with incomes below the federal poverty level ($10,284 for a family of three and $6,565 for a single person, as of 1992) are eligible. Medicaid eligibility has continuously fallen since it was first enacted, when 70 percent of those with incomes below the federal poverty level were eligible.

Those on Medicaid lose their eligibility once they become employed and their income rises above the Medicaid cutoff level, which could still be below the federal poverty level. The potential loss of their medical benefits is a disincentive for Medicaid recipients to accept low-paying jobs.

Medicaid patients' access to medical care has been reduced as states, to reduce their expenditures, have paid hospitals and physicians so little that health providers do not want to serve Medicaid patients.

Even with these restrictions on eligibility and provider payments, Medicaid has become a huge burden on state budgets. It is the fastest-growing state expenditure; in 1991, one-half of the states reported Medicaid expenditure increases of 20 percent or more. And unlike the federal government, states cannot incur a deficit; to fund increased Medicaid expenditures, they must either raise taxes or reduce funding for politically popular programs.

The Current State of Medicare

Medicare is a federal program that primarily serves the aged; those requiring kidney dialysis and transplants, regardless of age, were added in subsequent years. There are two parts to Medicare, Part A and Part B.

Part A

Part A covers acute hospital care, skilled nursing home care after hospitalization for rehabilitation, home health services, and hospice care for the terminally ill. All the aged are automatically enrolled in Part A when they retire at age 65. If a Medicare patient requires hospitalization they must pay a $676 deductible, as of 1993. The Medicare hospital trust fund (Part A) is financed by an earmarked Medicare Social Security Health Insurance (HI) tax, which, in 1966, was a combined .35 percent (.175 on both the employer and the employee) on wages up to $6,600. As Medicare expenditures exceeded projections, both the HI tax and the wage base on which the tax applied were increased. By 1986, the combined HI tax had risen to 1.45 percent on wages up to $42,000. Currently, the total HI tax is 2.90 percent on all earned income.

The Medicare Part A fund, which is used to pay for the hospital care incurred by current beneficiaries, is a "pay as you go" fund; current Medicare expenditures are funded by current employee and employer contributions. The HI taxes from current Medicare eligibles were never set aside for their own future expenses but were instead used to pay for those who were eligible at that time. This is in contrast to a pension fund, where a person sets aside funds to pay for his or her own retirement. Whenever the Medicare actuaries estimate that the trust fund will become insolvent—that is, current HI taxes are insufficient to pay current Medicare expenditures—Medicare HI taxes on employees and employers are increased.

In addition to increasing HI taxes to cover the expected shortfall, each administration has reduced its payments to hospitals for treating Medicare patients. As shown in Figure 8.2, when the DRG pricing system was introduced in the mid-1980s, and an annual limit was placed on the rise in the DRG price, the rate of increase in Medicare hospital expenditures (adjusted for inflation) per enrollee actually declined. Recently, expenditures for skilled nursing homes and home health care, which are included in Part A, increased by more than 40 percent, thereby causing total Part A expenditures to increase.

Part B

Medicare Part B is a supplemental medical insurance (SMI) program that covers physician and outpatient services. Those eligible for Medicare are not automatically enrolled in SMI; it is a voluntary program. However, more than 90 percent of the aged are willing to pay the $36.60 a month premium (as of 1993), which is a bargain since it covers only 25 percent of the program's costs. The remaining 75 percent of Part B expenditures are financed from federal tax revenues. The aged are responsible for an annual $100 deductible and a 20 percent copayment for their use of medical services.

Unlike the Medicare hospital trust fund, a crisis does not occur if Part B expenditures continually exceed projections; the federal deficit is merely increased. The growth in Part B expenditures has, however, become an important contributor to the current federal deficit. In 1992, the federal subsidy for Part B expenditures exceeded $50 billion. To limit the rise in these federal expenditures, a new physician pricing and

Figure 8.2   Growth in Real Medicare Expenditures per Enrollee,
Part A and Part B, 1966–1992

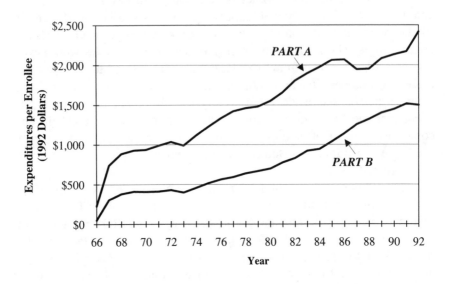

Note: Values adjusted for inflation using the consumer price index for all urban consumers.
Source: U.S. Department of Health and Human Services, Social Security Administration (Washington, DC), *Social Security Bulletin, Annual Statistical Supplement, 1993.*

expenditure control system (RBRVS) was implemented in 1992. As can be seen in Figure 8.2, it has had an effect on the growth in Part B expenditures.

"Medigap" Insurance

Almost 80 percent of the aged also purchase private "Medigap" insurance to cover their out-of-pocket costs (Parts A and B deductibles and the 20 percent Part B copayments), which can be substantial. Medigap policies provide the aged with nearly first-dollar coverage, which eliminates the constraints on unnecessary use of services that the copayments were designed to prevent.

Concerns

One concern with Medicare is that the benefits are the same for all the aged. Medicare pays, on average, only one-half of the aged's medical expenses; outpatient prescription drugs and long-term care are not covered. Also, those aged requiring home care or nursing home services, unrelated to an illness episode, must typically rely on their own funds to cover such expenses. Thus out-of-pocket payments for excluded benefits as a percent of income are very high for low-income aged, exceeding 20 percent, while, on average, it is less than 6 percent for high-income aged. Consequently, many low-income aged find the out-of-pocket expenses a financial hardship, and 8 percent must rely on Medicaid.

There are important differences between Medicare and Medicaid. Medicare is considered to be an "entitlement" program (the aged contributed HI taxes), as contrasted to Medicaid, which is a welfare program (the benefits have not been "earned"). Thus all the aged are eligible for Medicare, while income is used to determine eligibility for Medicaid. Medicaid is funded by general state and federal tax revenues; funding for Medicare is based on an earmarked Social Security HI tax (Part A) and federal tax revenues (Part B). How well these programs have served their respective beneficiaries, however, is more likely related to the populations they serve: The aged are politically powerful, whereas the poor are not. Therein lies the major reason for their differences.

How equitable is the financing of Medicare and Medicaid? Neither Medicare nor Medicaid beneficiaries pay the full costs of the medical services they receive; they are subsidized by those who pay state and federal taxes and Medicare HI taxes. The subsidy to Medicaid recipients is acknowledged to be "welfare," since they receive benefits in excess of any taxes they may have paid. Since Medicaid is a welfare program it is appropriately financed through the income tax system, whereby those with higher incomes contribute more, in both absolute and proportionate payments in relation to their income. This is the fairest way to finance a welfare program.

There is, however, a large "welfare" component to Medicare, since the aged's HI payments for Part A and their premium contributions for Part B have always been less than Medicare Part A and B expenditures on their behalf.

Medicare enrollees receive an intergenerational transfer of wealth (subsidy) from those currently in the labor force, which is no different from a conventional form of welfare. Several studies have estimated the difference between the present value of Medicare benefits received by the aged and the present value of the aged's HI taxes and Part B premium contributions. The difference between these benefits and contributions is the size of the intergenerational subsidy. For example, those aged who

Table 8.1 Money Income of Families, Percent Distribution by Income Quintile

Characteristic	Number (1,000)	Total	Percent Distribution					
			Lowest Fifth	Second Fifth	Third Fifth	Fourth Fifth	Highest Fifth	Top 5 Percent
15 to 24 years old	2,726	100.0	51.9	24.0	16.0	5.9	2.2	0.4
25 to 34 years old	14,590	100.0	24.1	21.8	22.1	20.4	11.7	1.8
35 to 44 years old	17,078	100.0	14.3	16.6	21.0	24.3	23.8	5.3
45 to 54 years old	11,701	100.0	11.2	13.9	18.2	23.4	33.4	9.0
55 to 64 years old	9,326	100.0	15.4	19.2	19.9	20.9	24.6	7.6
65 years old and over	10,900	100.0	28.9	29.2	18.6	12.0	11.3	3.4
65 to 74 years old	7,373	100.0	24.2	29.2	20.4	13.4	12.8	3.7
75 years old and over	3,527	100.0	38.6	29.4	14.8	9.1	8.1	2.7

Source: U.S. Bureau of the Census (Washington, DC), *Statistical Abstract of the United States, 1992*, Table No. 705, p. 450.

became eligible when Medicare was started in 1966 did not contribute anything into the Medicare HI trust fund. They received a 100 percent welfare subsidy. In subsequent years, as more aged became eligible, they made some contributions into the hospital trust fund, but it was too little to cover their Medicare costs. Vogel (1988) estimated that 95 percent of Medicare hospital expenditures in 1984 should be regarded as subsidies.

Iglehart (1992) states: "For those who retired in 1991, the current average value of a beneficiary's Medicare hospital benefit far exceeds his or her contribution: $5.09 of services has been paid for under Part A for every $1 contributed. The ratio of benefits to contributions is even greater for people who retired earlier." To these Part A subsidies should be added the 75 percent federal subsidy for Part B premiums, which exceeded $50 billion in 1992.

To determine whether the subsidy provided to Medicare beneficiaries is equitably financed, it is necessary to examine the incomes of the beneficiaries and of those who bear the cost. As shown in Table 8.1, incomes are highest in the 45–54 age group. However, the aged have a similar income distribution to those in the 25–34 group. There is a difference among the aged, with those 65–74 having much higher incomes than those 75 and older. The incomes of the aged are understated relative to the non-aged because the aged pay only 13 percent of their income in taxes, compared to 23 percent for all ages. Over 75 percent of the aged own their own homes, and about three-fourths of those do not owe any mortgage; thus some form of imputed rent on these homes would substantially increase the incomes of the aged. Also, the aged receive many in-kind subsidies, such as Medicare, housing, and subsidized meal programs, the value of which is not shown as part of their reported income. If the incomes of the aged were adjusted for these differences, many aged would have higher incomes than many non-aged.

Since the Medicare subsidy is available to all the aged, regardless of their incomes, and their subsidy is financed from all employees, an inequitable situation arises. Lower-income employees are taxed to subsidize the medical expenses of higher-income Medicare eligibles.

Payroll taxes, which are used to fund Part A, are not a desirable method of financing a "welfare" program. While the employer and the employee each pay one-half of the Medicare HI tax, the reality is that the employee effectively bears most of the employer's share of the tax as well. When an employer decides how many employees to hire and what wage to pay, they consider all the costs of that employee. Any tax or regulatory cost imposed on the employer, based on their number of employees, is the same as requiring the employer to pay higher wages to those employees. It does not matter to the employer whether the cost of that employee is in the form of wages, fringe benefits, or taxes; it is a cost of labor. An increase in the employer's HI tax increases the cost of labor.

When the cost of an employee is increased and exceeds their value to the employer, the employer will discharge the employee, unless they can reduce the employee's wages so the cost does not exceed the employee's value. What typically occurs when payroll taxes are increased is wages are eventually renegotiated. Employees receive less than they would otherwise have received because of higher Social Security taxes imposed on the employer. Thus most of the employer's share of the tax is shifted to the employee in the form of lower wages. Studies confirm that employees end up paying most of the employer's share of the Social Security tax (Brittain 1971).

A tax per employee, imposed on the employer, rarely stays with the employer. Even though the employer pays the tax, it is usually shifted back to the employee in the form of lower wages. That part of the tax not shifted back to the employee will be shifted forward in the form of higher prices for goods and services. For example, most industries are competitive and do not earn excessive profits; otherwise, firms would enter the industry and compete away those profits. When the HI tax is increased on both the employee and employer, employment contracts cannot be immediately renegotiated. Rather than being forced to reduce its profits and leave the industry, the employer will shift the tax forward to the consumer by raising prices. Whether the tax is shifted back to the employee or forward to the consumer, the tax is *regressive*; those with low incomes pay a greater portion of their income in Social Security taxes than do higher-income people. Only recently has the HI tax become proportional to wages; since interest and dividend income is excluded from the tax, only a portion of an employee's income is subject to the tax. When the tax is passed on to the consumer, the higher prices are a greater proportionate burden on low-income consumers.

Since the tax is shifted either forward or backward, why is one-half of the tax imposed on the employer? The reason is related more to its visibility than who ends up paying it. Politicians would prefer to make employees believe their share is much smaller than it actually is.

If society makes the value judgment that it wants to help those with low incomes by providing them with a welfare benefit, the most equitable way to do so would be to provide the majority of benefits to those with low incomes and finance those benefits by taxing those with higher incomes. The burden of financing Medicare Part A, however, has fallen more heavily on those with lower incomes. Many aged who receive Part A medical benefits have higher incomes and assets than those who are providing the subsidies, as shown in Table 8.1. An income tax, which takes proportionately more from those with higher incomes, would be a more equitable way to finance benefits to those with low incomes. While the investment and retirement income of high-income aged are not subject to payroll taxes, they are subject to income taxes.

The Future of Medicare and Medicaid

Medicare and Medicaid should be changed. The Medicare HI trust fund is expected to be bankrupt by 1998. Each time the trust fund approaches insolvency, HI taxes and the wage base are increased and hospital payments are decreased. Over the long term, however, these approaches to staving off bankruptcy cannot be successful because the aged are growing, both in numbers and as a portion of the population. In 1980, approximately 11 percent of the population, or 26 million people, were 65 years and older. By 2030, the number of aged are expected to increase to 66 million, or 22 percent of the population. The employee base for supporting Medicare is eroding; there are fewer workers per aged person today, and this ratio will become worse over time.

The 1990 report of the Medicare Part A Board of Trustees estimated that Medicare payroll taxes would have to rise from the current 2.9 percent to more than 4 percent by the year 2010 and to more than 7 percent of payroll by 2030 if the trust fund is to remain solvent. The political support for Medicare is likely to decline as the costs to the non-aged increase. Intergenerational conflict is likely to occur.

The federal commitment to fund Part B benefits is open-ended. The increase in the number of aged and in their use of Part B services requires the federal government to pay 75 percent of those costs, regardless of their magnitude, and the large and growing federal subsidies to Part B (in excess of $50 billion in 1992) further contribute to the federal deficit.

Rising Medicare and Medicaid expenditures are increasing the financial pressure on the federal and state governments to bring about a new political solution. The "entitlement" myth of Medicare must be recognized and its large welfare component acknowledged if meaningful changes are to be made. Making Medicare benefits income-related would reduce both the cost of the program and the perverse intergenerational subsidy that occurs when low-income workers subsidize high-income aged. Income-related benefits would also help the low-income aged, who are less able to afford the same deductibles, cost-sharing, and Part B premiums than high-income aged.

Medicare benefits can be made income-related by providing the aged with a voucher for a uniform set of benefits in a managed care organization. The value of the voucher would equal the entire premium for low-income aged and would decline in value the higher the income of the aged. As a transition to this approach, all current aged could receive the full value of the voucher. The income-related voucher would be phased in for future aged.

Medicaid should be similarly replaced with an income-related voucher for all persons with low incomes. By only losing a portion of their voucher as their income rose, those with low incomes would no longer have a disincentive to accept low-paying jobs.

The income-related approach, in addition to improving equity, would also improve efficiency, since managed care plans would compete for the vouchers. Neither Medicare nor Medicaid include sufficient incentives for program efficiency. Both programs rely on fee-for-service, and both physicians and patients have incentives to "overuse" medical services. Medical services are virtually free to those on Medicaid, and "Medigap" insurance eliminates patients' cost concerns. Medicare eligibles have limited financial incentives to limit their use of services or to join managed care systems. Only about 10 percent of Medicare and Medicaid eligibles are enrolled in HMOs. If the states were to contract with managed care organizations for their Medicaid population, more efficient use of services would occur and Medicaid patients would receive better access to providers.

Although the federal government pays HMOs 95 percent of the aged's average Part A and Part B costs when the HMO enrolls an aged beneficiary, the government has determined that they still lose money when the aged join HMOs. Apparently HMOs receive, on average, a favorable risk group of aged enrollees; that is, 95 percent of the average aged's costs is greater than what those aged in HMOs would have cost had they not been in HMOs. For the government to save money on Medicare HMOs, it will be necessary to develop risk-adjusted premiums. The ability of the aged to disenroll from the HMO after one month's notice should also be changed to a one year "lock-in" to prevent preferred-risk selection.

When Congress enacted the Medicare Catastrophic Act in 1989, high-income aged were required to increase their Part B contributions to finance greater benefits to low-income aged. The protests of the high-income aged were so great that Congress repealed the legislation. This attempt at increased fairness failed and will make it more difficult for Congress to enact equitable Medicare reform. However, the longer it takes to phase in a system that is more equitably financed and relates benefits to income, the greater will be the intergenerational transfers from low-income workers and the longer will be the financial hardship on low-income aged who cannot afford high out-of-pocket expenditures.

References

Brittain, J. A. "The Incidence of Social Security Payroll Taxes." *American Economic Review* 61 (March 1971): 110–25.
Iglehart, J. K. "The American Health Care System—Introduction." *New England Journal of Medicine* 326 (2 April 1992): 966.
Vogel, R. J. "An Analysis of the Welfare Component and Intergenerational Transfers under the Medicare Program." In *Lessons from the First Twenty Years of Medicare*, edited by M. V. Pauly and W. L. Kissick. Philadelphia: University of Pennsylvania Press, 1988.

9

The New Medicare
Physician Payment System

In 1992 a radical new payment system for physician services under Medicare began to be phased in over a five-year period. Why was it necessary to change to a new system? How does the new payment system compare to the previous one? And what are likely to be the effects of this new payment system on access to care by Medicare patients, on physician fees paid by the non-aged working population, and on physicians' incomes?

The Previous System

When Medicare was enacted in 1965, Part B was included, which paid for physician and out-of-hospital services. Physicians were paid fee-for-service for Medicare patients and were given the choice of whether or not to be a participating physician (or even whether to participate for some medical claims but not others). When physicians participated, they agreed to accept the Medicare fee for that service and the patient was responsible for only 20 percent of that fee, after they paid their annual deductible.

If the physician was not a participating physician, then the patient would have to pay the physician's entire charge, which was higher than the Medicare fee, and apply for reimbursement from Medicare. When the government reimbursed the patient, however, they would only pay the patient 80 percent of the Medicare-approved fee for that service.

Thus a patient going to a nonparticipating physician would have to pay 20 percent of the physician's Medicare-approved fee, plus the difference between the approved fee and the physician's actual charges. This difference is referred to as *balance billing*. Medicare patients going to nonparticipating physicians were also burdened by the paperwork of sending their bills to Medicare for reimbursement.

As physicians' fees and Medicare expenditures rapidly increased, the government placed a limit on physicians' Medicare fees in 1972, referred to as the Medicare Economic Index. Physicians' fees, however, continued to increase sharply in the private sector, and as the difference between private physician fees and the Medicare-approved fee became larger, fewer physicians chose to participate in Medicare. Consequently, more of the aged were balance-billed the difference between their physician's fee and the Medicare-approved fee.

Medicare fee-for-service payment also encouraged greater use of services. As limits were placed on participating physicians' fees, there was concern that physicians encouraged more visits and engaged in more testing to increase their Medicare billings ("induced demand"). Even with limits on physicians' fees, Medicare Part B expenditures continued to increase rapidly, as shown previously in Figure 8.2.

Reasons for Adoption of the New System

The new Medicare physician payment system was adopted for three reasons. The most important was the federal government's desire to limit the rise in the federal budget deficit. Expenditures under Medicare Part B, 75 percent of which are for physicians' services—the remainder are for other, nonhospital services—have been increasing rapidly, at approximately 10 percent per year. Part B expenditures reached $50 billion in 1992 and are expected to go as high as $70 billion a year by 1996. As Medicare physician payments continue to rise, the government's portion, 75 percent of the total, contributes directly to the growing federal budget deficit. Both Republican and Democratic administrations believed that if the government was to reduce the size of the federal deficit, the growth in Part B expenditures must be slowed.

Second, many physicians and academicians believed that the previous Medicare payment system was inequitable. A new physician first establishing a fee schedule with Medicare could receive higher fees than an older physician whose fee increases were limited by the Medicare

Economic Index. Physicians who performed procedures, for example, diagnostic testing and surgery, were paid at a much higher rate per unit of physician time than were physicians who performed cognitive services, such as office examinations. Also, Medicare fees for the same procedure varied greatly across geographic areas, unrelated to differences in practice costs.

The aged were also expected to benefit from the new payment system by limiting increases in their out-of-pocket expense. They would no longer be balance-billed, and their annual Part B premium would not increase very rapidly since the government will control the overall rate of growth in physician expenditures.

Components of the New System

Reducing the federal deficit by limiting Part B expenditures, achieving greater Medicare fee equity among physicians, and limiting the aged's payments led to the three main parts of the physician payment reform package.

Resource-Based Relative Value Scale Fee Schedule

The first, and most publicized, is the creation of a Resource-Based Relative Value Scale (RBRVS) fee schedule. Three resource components were used to construct the fee for a particular service. The first, the work component, was an estimate of the cost of providing a particular service, including the time, intensity, skill, and mental effort and stress involved in providing the service. Second is the physician's practice expenses, such as salaries and rent. Third is malpractice insurance. Each component is assigned a relative value; the greater the costs and time required for a service, the higher was the relative value unit (RVU). A procedure with a value of 20 is believed to be twice as costly as one with a value of 10.

The actual fee was then determined by multiplying these relative value units by a conversion factor, which is politically determined. For example, "transplantation of the heart" is assigned 44.13 work RVUs, 49.24 practice expense RVUs, and 9.17 malpractice RVUs, for a total of 102.54 RVUs. The 1992 conversion factor was $31, making the fee for this procedure $3,178 ($31 × 102.54). This fee is then adjusted for geographic location.

RBRVS reduces the variation in fees both within the same specialty and across geographic regions. New physicians receive 80 percent of the Medicare fee schedule in their first year, with the percentage rising to 100 percent by the fifth year. Medicare fees will still vary geographically by 12 percent less and 18 percent more than the average, but this is greatly reduced from the previous geographic variation. As a result, California physicians will have their fees reduced by 14 percent, while fees in Mississippi will be increased by 11 percent.

The new payment system reflects the cost of performing 7,000 different physician services. When constructing the RBRVS fee structure, Professor William Hsiao of Harvard found that physician fees were not closely related to the resource costs needed to produce those services. In general, "cognitive" services, such as patient evaluation, counseling, and management of services, were greatly undervalued compared with procedural services, such as surgery and testing. RBRVS reduces the profitability of procedures while increasing payment for cognitive services. By changing the relative weights of different types of services, the RBRVS system will cause substantial shifts in payments, and consequently incomes, among physicians. In large metropolitan areas, for example, payments to surgeons would decline by 25 percent. The "winners" and "losers" among physician specialties are shown in Figure 9.1.

Volume-Expenditure Limit

The RBRVS approach is still, however, fee-for-service payment and by itself does not control the volume of services nor total physician expenditures. Because the government was concerned that physicians would induce demand to offset their lower Medicare fees, the second part of the new payment system is a limit on overall physician Medicare expenditures. This limit is achieved by linking the annual update on physician fees (the conversion factor) to the growth in volume of services. If volume increases more rapidly than a target rate, which is based on increases in inflation, number of beneficiaries, newly covered services, and technological advances, then Congress will reduce the annual fee update the following year. Too rapid an increase in services will result in a smaller fee update.

Balance-Billing Limit

The third part of the new payment system, in addition to the RBRVS fee schedule and the volume-expenditure limit, is a limit (and a virtual phasing out) on the amount that physicians are able to balance-bill Medicare patients.

Figure 9.1   Medicare Physician Fee Schedule, Effect on Fees by
Specialty, 1992

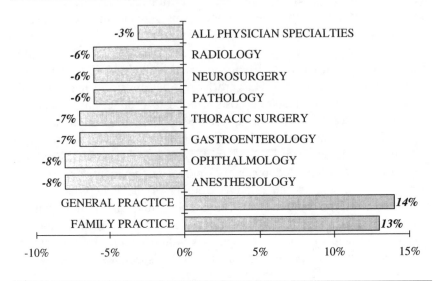

Source: "Medicare Physician Payment Reform Regulations," Hearing before the U.S. Senate Subcommittee on Medicare and Long-Term Care of the Committee on Finance, 19 July 1991.

Effects of the New Payment System

To analyze the likely effects of the new payment system, let us initially assume that physicians do *not* induce demand; that is, as these new fees reduce specialists' incomes, physicians are not motivated to manipulate the patient's demand (for a more complete discussion of the effects of the new physician payment system, see Frech 1991 and Pauly 1992).

RBRVS will reduce fees for procedures, such as surgery, while increasing fees for cognitive services. With lower fees for surgery, for example, we might expect surgeons to perform fewer Medicare surgeries, since they could reallocate their time to performing surgeries for private patients, whose fees were not reduced. However, if surgeons are not as busy as they would prefer and the Medicare fee still exceeds the value of their time spent doing nonsurgical tasks, surgeons will not reduce their Medicare surgeries and will continue to perform the same number of procedures. The effect of lower fees for procedures with no change in the number of procedures will result in a decrease in Medicare procedure-type expenditures and lower specialists' incomes.

What about specialists' private patients? Would their fees be increased to make up for lower Medicare fees? Physicians allocate their time between two markets: Medicare and non-Medicare (private) patients. Specialists' fees for private patients are presumably already at their highest level, consistent with making as much profit as possible from those patients. If they are not charging as much as the market would bear, why aren't they, since they would be forgoing income they could have earned? If private fees were increased further (beyond what the market would bear), the loss in revenue from lower volume would exceed the gain in revenue from those higher fees. The specialist would be worse off. (See Chapter 14, on cost shifting.) The specialist might be able to increase his or her volume from private-pay patients by decreasing the fee to such patients. Lowering the fee would be a more profitable strategy than raising it if the gain in revenue from increased volume more than offset the loss in revenues from decreased fees.

Assume that before Medicare lowered its fees, the specialist was allocating his or her time between private and Medicare patients so that the profit from each type of patient was the same. Once Medicare reduces its fees, the profit per hour of the specialist's time becomes greater serving private patients. The specialist should serve fewer Medicare patients and more private patients. However, the only way the specialist could serve more private patients is to reduce their fees. Thus it is unlikely that the specialist would want to or be able to "cost shift" to private patients.

If the specialist has excess capacity and does not attempt to induce demand, then the aged would have no less access than previously, specialists would provide the same volume of services, they would suffer reduced incomes, and Medicare expenditures for specialist services would decline.

Physicians who are willing to "create" demand to offset declines in their incomes would first attempt to induce demand among their private patients. A greater volume of private patients would be more profitable since the private fee has not been reduced. Only then would the specialist create demand among the Medicare patients, whose fees have been reduced. But if specialists are not busy enough, then it is likely that they have already tried to induce as much demand as possible and would be unable to induce much further demand. Instead they might engage in such fraudulent practices as "code creep," which is a way of increasing their Medicare fee.

Medicare expenditures and specialist incomes would still be expected to decline among physicians inclined to induce demand, assuming that these specialists previously had excess capacity. To the extent that demand inducers are able to engage in code creep, they will be able to offset some of the decline in their incomes. If specialists were fully busy, then the reductions in Medicare specialist fees would result in a reallocation of their time to private patients (whose fees are higher) and, consequently, reduced access by Medicare patients.

Under RBRVS, Medicare fees for cognitive services will be increased, which will cause primary care physicians to reallocate their time to where their profit per hour is greater. Since the higher fees increase the profitability of Medicare patients, primary care physicians would be expected to serve more Medicare patients and fewer private patients. As physicians decrease their available time to private patients, and private demand will exceed the available physician time for private patients, fees for private patients should increase. Total Medicare expenditures for cognitive services, particularly for primary care physicians, will increase.

Primary care physicians who may have been willing to induce demand to increase their incomes might be less inclined to do so, since their incomes will increase as a result of their fee increases. Those who are still inclined to induce demand will find it more profitable to do so for their Medicare patients, whose fees have increased, and less so for their private patients.

What will be the overall effect on expenditures as a result of the new fee schedule? Assuming specialists are not busy enough, little additional demand inducement will be possible and the result will be lower Medicare Part B expenditures. While expenditures will increase for primary care physicians, whose fees have increased, these increases are likely to be less than the decreases in specialist expenditures. As shown by the recent change in trend in Part B expenditures in Figure 8.2, this is apparently what has occurred.

The volume-expenditure limit, which is part of the RBRVS system, was meant to control demand inducement. If specialists already have excess capacity, then demand inducement of additional procedures is likely to be small. Specialists may attempt to induce some demand for their cognitive services (whose fees have increased), but this is likely to have a small effect since it is not a large part of their practice.

Over time, however, Medicare physician expenditures will continue to increase because of inflation, growth in the aged population, and new technologies. Unless Congress permits the volume-expenditure limit to reflect these pressures for higher expenditures, shortages could result. As demands for care by both Medicare and private patients increase, primary care physicians will attempt to increase their fees, since primary care physicians are less likely to have excess capacity. To the extent that Medicare fee increases match fee increases to private patients, the physician would not find it profitable to change their allocation of time to each group of patients. But if volume increases because of an increase in the number of beneficiaries, and Congress, to save money, limits Medicare fee increases, the relative profitability of Medicare patients would decline.

Only by "raising" their Medicare fee by such methods as reducing the time spent per Medicare visit and having the patient return more often, thereby creating multiple visits for what was previously done in one visit, would it be profitable for primary care physicians to continue seeing the same number of Medicare patients.

Greater fee increases for private patients will cause physicians to reallocate their time to such patients. Medicare patients would then have less access to primary care physicians. However, if physicians were able to balance-bill their Medicare patients, then relative fees between Medicare and private patients would remain the same and the physician would not reallocate his or her time away from Medicare patients. The inability of primary care physicians to balance-bill will result in shortages of physician services for Medicare patients; the demand for such services will exceed the amount physicians are willing to supply at the lower Medicare fee.

Limiting balance-billing and establishing a uniform fee schedule among physicians (within the same specialty) has another unfortunate effect. Previously, differences in fees for the same service may have reflected differences in that service. For example, some physicians are of higher quality, while others may spend more time listening to the patient's concerns. Although the service may be nominally similar, the content of that service may differ. In the above examples, the costs of providing that service, in terms of the physician's time, differs. Patients are willing to pay more for certain attributes of their physicians, such as their ability to relate to the patient. By having a uniform fee schedule with virtually no balance-billing, the physician treating Medicare patients is unable to charge for these extra attributes. Busy primary care physicians could provide additional visits and earn a higher income instead of spending time on these extra attributes.

The new RBRVS national fee schedule, with volume-expenditure controls and limits on balance-billing, was an attempt to limit federal expenditures for Medicare physician services, to improve equity among different medical specialties, and to limit out-of-pocket payments and Part B premiums by the aged. Medicare expenditures will, however, continue to rise as the number of eligible aged increase, along with inflation, and advances in technology, which makes possible the provision of new services for the aged. The demands for some physician specialties, such as primary care, will grow faster than other specialties. Congress is unlikely to be able to accurately forecast the "right" rate of increase in Medicare expenditures because they are more likely to be concerned with limiting the rise in Medicare expenditures than in properly adjusting for changes in the number of aged, inflation, and technology. The consequences to the aged of "too slow" an increase in Medicare expenditures will be a shortage of primary care services.

A uniform fee schedule cannot indicate that a shortage is developing in some areas or among certain physician specialties. Similarly, uniform fees cannot eliminate such shortages. Unless a national fee schedule is flexible, allowing fees for some services, physicians, and geographic regions to increase more rapidly than others, shortages will arise and persist. Permitting physicians to balance-bill their Medicare patients would indicate that an imbalance between demand and supply has occurred. The government could then raise fees in those areas and among those specialties where balance-billing is increasing.

Fees provide information; they signal that changes have occurred in either the costs of providing care or in the demands for that care or both. If the government does not want to overpay specialties and services that are in oversupply, while underpaying those that are in short supply, a flexible mechanism, such as balance-billing, is needed. Otherwise, the aged will find that they have reduced access to care, and the government will not be spending its money wisely.

References

Frech III, H. E., ed. *Regulating Doctors' Fees: Competition, Benefits and Controls under Medicare.* Washington, DC: AEI Press, 1991.

Pauly, M. V., J. M. Eisenberg, M. H. Radany, M. H. Erder, R. Feldman, and J. J. Schwartz. *Paying Physicians: Options for Controlling Cost, Volume, and Intensity of Services.* Ann Arbor, Michigan: Health Administration Press, 1992.

10

Physician Incomes

Major changes have been occurring in the market for physicians' services. There has been a large increase in the supply of physicians, from 311,203 in 1970, to 435,545 in 1980, to 615,421 in 1990. The antitrust laws were held to be applicable to the health field. Preferred provider organizations (PPOs) formed and selected physicians based on their willingness to discount their fees. Managed care organizations, which include HMOs and indemnity plans that use utilization review, became the norm rather than the exception and questioned physicians on their prescribing patterns, such as their use of the hospital and certain surgical procedures. Outpatient diagnostics and surgery greatly increased as a result of technological changes and payment incentives. The federal government instituted a new physician payment system for Medicare patients. These market changes are affecting both physician incomes and their practices.

Supply and Demand for Physicians

Physician incomes are determined by the interplay of supply and demand. If the demand for physicians increases more rapidly than the number of physicians, physician incomes will increase. Conversely, if the supply of physicians has been rising more rapidly than demand, physician incomes will rise less rapidly (or fall, once adjusted for inflation).

At the beginning of the 1980s, median physician incomes (i.e., the 50th percentile) declined, then rose during the latter part of the decade.[1]

Over the entire decade of the 1980s, median physician incomes increased faster than inflation and rose on average 2.1 percent (net of inflation) per year, from $75,000 in 1981 to $130,000 in 1990 (see Figure 10.1).

The data presented in Figure 10.1 are averages based on all physicians. Certain physician specialties fared much better than others, as shown in Figure 10.2. Physicians in surgical specialties, such as cardiology and orthopedics, and radiology received the largest annual increases in incomes (3.6 percent and 4.2 percent, inflation adjusted) compared to those in general and family practice (0.4 percent annually). Those specialties that had the largest incomes were also those who benefited most during the 1980s. In 1991, median incomes were lowest for general/family practice physicians ($111,000), compared to those in surgical specialties ($233,000). As discussed below, those physician specialties who were able to benefit from new diagnostic and surgical techniques were also those with the highest incomes and the largest annual percent increases in their incomes.

To understand the rise in physician incomes during the 1980s,

Figure 10.1   Annual Percent Changes in Median Physician Net Income after Expenses before Taxes, 1982–1991

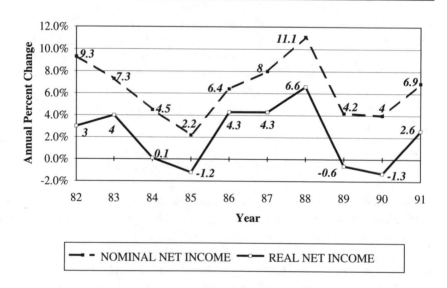

Source: American Medical Association, Center for Health Policy Studies (Chicago, IL), *Socioeconomic Characteristics of Medical Practice, 1993.*

Figure 10.2 Average Annual Percent Change in Mean Real Net Income of Self-Employed Physicians by Specialty, 1981–1991

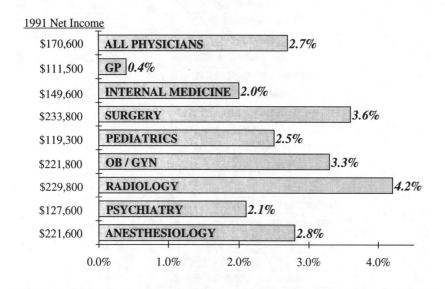

Note: Values were adjusted for inflation using the consumer price index for all urban consumers. GP = General and family practice.

Sources: American Medical Association (Chicago, IL), *Socioeconomic Characteristics of Medical Practice, 1989 and 1993 editions.*

it becomes necessary to understand why the demand for physicians exceeded the supply of physicians.

Between 1970 and 1980, the number of physicians per 100,000 population increased by 25 percent, from 161 per 100,000 to 202 per 100,000, as shown in Figure 4.1. The number of physicians in relation to the population continued to expand during the 1980s, but at a slower rate of increase. Between 1980 and 1985, the physician to population ratio continued to expand at a 2.5 percent annual rate. However, during the last five years of the 1980s, supply increased at one-half that rate, 1.4 percent annually.

Although there have been large increases in the supply of physicians, the demand for physicians has been increasing more rapidly. In addition to rising physician incomes, increased physician fees are another indication of greater relative increases in demand. Physician fees, however, could also rise for another reason: the cost of providing physician

Figure 10.3   Annual Percent Changes in the Consumer Price Index and in Physicians' Fees, 1965–1992

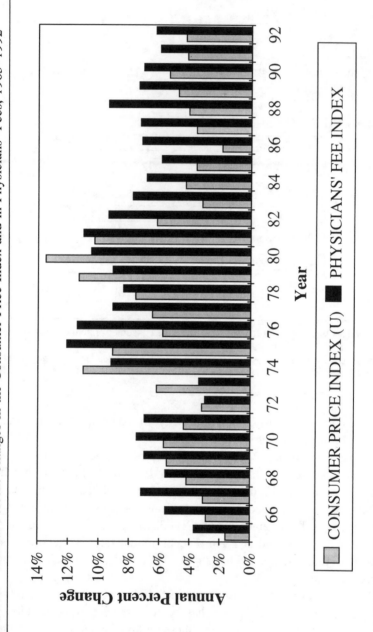

Note: CPI (U) = consumer price index for all urban consumers.
Sources: U.S. Bureau of the Census (Washington, DC), *Statistical Abstract of the United States* and *Historical Abstract of the United States,* various editions.

services, such as higher office expenses, employee wages, and malpractice premiums could increase. These higher costs would also cause physicians to raise their fees. Regardless of whether higher costs are the reason for increasing fees, they are always used as the justification. Few physicians or businesses would claim that because demand has increased they are increasing their prices so as to make a greater profit. Instead, it is more socially acceptable to justify higher prices by citing higher costs.

To illustrate that the higher fees are more the result of demand rising faster than supply rather than higher costs of physician services, Figure 10.3 shows increases in physician fees relative to the consumer price index (CPI). While the CPI is not a perfect measure of the costs of providing physician services, it provides a rough approximation of how wage costs are changing, which are the major portion of a physician's office expenses. The growth in malpractice premiums, which had been rising at 29 percent per year in the early 1980s, slowed to less than 4 percent per year by the late 1980s; malpractice premiums, however, represent only 10 percent of physician office expenses.

Physician fees increased at a much more rapid rate than the CPI during the mid-1980s, and while fees are still rising faster than the CPI, their difference is smaller. One reason for the less rapid rate of increase in physician fees is the recent recession. During the late 1970s and early 1980s, the previous recession, physician fees actually declined (relative to the CPI).

Total expenditures on physician services include both fee increases and changes in volume of services. When adjusted for the increased number of physicians, the growth in expenditures per physician is the same as gross revenue received per physician. As shown in Table 10.1, throughout the 1970s and 1980s, physician expenditures were increasing between 15 to 20 percent per year. On a per physician basis (to adjust for the greater number of physicians), expenditures (gross revenues) per physician have been increasing between 9 to 12 percent per year.

Since inflation was higher in the 1970s than the 1980s, physician gross revenues are adjusted for inflation. When "real" gross revenues per physician are compared to the average percent increase in "real" physician fees, we observe that during the 1970s both increased at a very slow rate per year, suggesting that physician incomes also increased slowly during that period. During the 1980s, particularly from 1985 to 1990, physician incomes increased more rapidly, and most of the annual increase in physician incomes resulted from real fee increases (3.4 percent per year) rather than increased number of services.

Table 10.1   Annual Percent Changes in Physician Expenditures, Fees, and Inflation, 1965–1991

	1965	1970	1980	1985	1990	1991
Physician expenditures						
($ billions)	8.2	13.6	41.9	74.0	128.8	142.0
Average annual % change		13.2%	20.8%	15.3%	14.8%	10.2%
Expenditures per physician						
($ thousands)	29.5	43.7	96.2	144.8	209.3	223.6
Average annual % change		9.6%	12.0%	10.1%	8.9%	6.8%
"Real" expenditures per physician (1991 $ thousands)	127.6	153.4	159.0	183.3	218.1	223.6
Average annual % change		4.0%	0.4%	3.1%	3.8%	2.5%
Annual % change in physician fees		7.5%	12.2%	9.6%	8.4%	6.0%
Annual % change in the consumer price index		4.6%	11.2%	6.1%	4.3%	4.2%
Average annual % change in "real" physician fees		2.3%	0.4%	2.7%	3.4%	1.8%

Note: Annual percent changes are author's calculations.
Sources: Health Care Financing Administration, Office of National Health Statistics (Baltimore, MD), and U.S. Department of Commerce, Bureau of the Census (Washington, DC), *Statistical Abstract of the United States*, various editions.

Reasons for Increases in Physician Expenditures and Incomes

There are several reasons why physician expenditures and incomes increased over time, but the importance of these reasons differed between the 1970s and the 1980s.

Demographics

Population has steadily increased by about 1 percent per year since the 1960s. The aging of the population, which uses more medical services, has, however, been a more important reason for increased demands for physician services. Since 1966, a Medicare patient had to pay a small annual deductible and then a 20 percent copayment when they went to the physician. This reduction in the price charged to the aged (20 percent of the fee) led to increased use of physician services and made them less price sensitive to the physician's charges. Because of rapid annual increases in physician fees to Medicare patients (80 percent of which is paid for by Medicare), the government in the early 1970s limited physicians' fee increases to Medicare patients. As Medicare limited physician fee increases, the aged's out-of-pocket copayment, on an inflation-adjusted basis, fell. This reduction in price faced by the aged further stimulated their demand for physician services.

Private Insurance

The growth in private insurance also reduced the out-of-pocket price faced by private patients. As shown in Figure 10.4, consumer direct payments for physician services, which was 63 percent in 1960, fell to 43 percent by 1970, after the enactment of Medicare and Medicaid. The public portion increased from 7 percent to 22 percent over that same time period. By 1991, consumers were only paying 18 percent of physician expenditures out-of-pocket, while private insurance and government increased to 47 percent and 35 percent, respectively. As patients' out-of-pocket payments for physician services declined, their demand increased, they became less price sensitive to what physicians were charging, and physician fees rose sharply.

Medical Technology

The growth in medical technology during the 1980s, particularly in outpatient settings, stimulated demand for these procedures, which were paid for by Medicare and private insurance. As new diagnostic and surgical procedures were developed, high fees were established to reflect the large number of hours specialists initially had to devote to performing these new procedures, such as cataract operations, coronary bypass surgery, and endoscopies. As physicians gained experience with these procedures, they were able to spend less time performing a specific procedure and performed additional procedures. These productivity gains should have been reflected in a lowering of fees. However, in the regulated environment in which fees were established by government for Medicare patients and by insurance companies for non-Medicare patients, fees were not reduced. Thus as the physician's cost (time) of performing the procedure fell and fees for new diagnostic and surgical procedures did not, these procedures became very profitable relative to the physician's time investment.

Figure 10.4   Percent Distribution of Physician Expenditures by
Source of Funds, Selected Years, 1960–1991

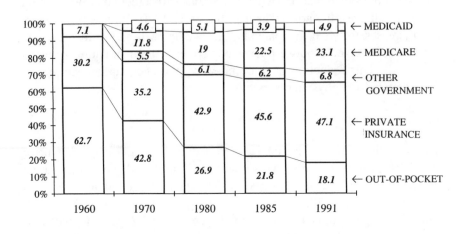

Source: S. W. Letsch, H. C. Lazenby, K. R. Levit, C. A. Cowan, "National Health
Expenditures, 1991," *Health Care Financing Review* 14 (Winter 1992): 1–29.

Thus part of the rapid increase in physician fees was a result of
changes in the types of physician services being provided. The increase
in the proportion of physicians that are specialists, together with new
technology, changed the composition of physician services that patients
were receiving. More expensive diagnostic and surgical procedures raised
average fees. The high volume of these surgical procedures, particularly
in outpatient settings during the 1980s, and physician productivity gains
in performing these procedures resulted in procedure-oriented specialists
receiving much higher profit margins per hour than physicians in primary
care, who performed few procedures.

The Future for Physician Incomes

Changes that are occurring in the physician marketplace are making
it unlikely that the trends in incomes for specialists will continue into
the 1990s.

The growth in managed care systems, including HMOs and PPOs,
that has been occurring since the mid-1980s has increased competition

among the increasing supply of physicians and is changing the structure of medical practice. To avoid losing patients, physicians are participating in these alternative delivery systems, discounting their fees, and accepting utilization review. Further, the number of physicians joining medical groups has increased, as has the size of the group. Although most physicians in group practice are in single-specialty groups, multispecialty groups are larger in size (24 physicians on average compared to 10 in single-specialty groups) and are increasing in size more rapidly than single-specialty groups.

The growth in medical groups has been driven by economies of scale in medical practice and by physicians' attempts to increase their market power. The administrative costs of running an office (including making appointments; billing patients, government, and insurance companies for services rendered; computerized information systems to keep track of patients) as well as use of aides to assist the physician, do not increase proportionately as the number of physicians increase. Larger group practices are also able to receive volume discounts on supplies and negotiate lower rentals on their leases than can the same number of physicians practicing separately or in smaller groups. The greater the number of physicians in a group, the lower will be their administrative and practice costs per physician.

Large medical groups are able to bid for HMO contracts and serve as a PPO provider for employers and insurers. Their size enables an insurer or an HMO to negotiate with one physician organization rather than have separate, time-consuming negotiations with a large number of individual physicians. Thus large medical groups are better able than individual physicians and smaller medical groups to compete for patients. An employer or insurer contracting with a large medical group has less reason to be concerned with physician quality. Large medical groups have more formalized quality control and monitoring mechanisms than do large numbers of independently practicing physicians. Within a large group, physicians refer to their own specialists; thus unless a specialist is part of a group they are less likely to have access to patients. These contracting, quality review, and referral mechanisms provide physicians within large medical groups with a competitive advantage over physicians unaffiliated with such groups.

Large multispecialty groups must have about two-thirds of their physicians in primary care, compared to about one-third in the current physician population. The movement toward capitation payments to providers requires a large number of primary care physicians to care for the insured population and for the primary care physician to be the gatekeeper to the use of specialists. Control over access to specialists is essential for controlling medical expenditures, which is of particular concern to medical groups who are at risk under capitation contracts. The specialists are the ones who order most of the tests, perform the procedures, and hospitalize the patients.

The emergence of primary care based multispecialty groups is a natural response by physicians to capitation-based competition. Specialists will become dependent upon primary care physicians for their referrals. Specialists who are unaffiliated with large multispecialty groups will find it more difficult to receive referrals from these groups. As specialist referrals become more tightly controlled by primary care physicians and the number of specialists needed under capitation falls, there is likely to be a growing surplus of specialists.

Multispecialty medical groups are increasing in size, and many are as large as 250 physicians. These groups are large economic entities. They are large enough to bear the risk themselves of being paid on a capitation contract with HMOs, and because they refer a large number of patients for hospitalization, they have a great deal of leverage when negotiating with hospitals.

Unless hospitals are affiliated with these large medical groups, they will have to compete among themselves for the medical group's hospital referrals. As admission rates continue to decline, there will be an even larger surplus of hospital capacity. Hospitals will be forced to deeply discount their rates, and even then they might not survive. It is for this reason that many hospitals are seeking to affiliate and even purchase medical groups. Again, the most valuable types of physicians for which hospitals are recruiting are those in primary care.

As the demand by large multispecialty medical groups for primary care physicians increases, so should their incomes, relative to specialists. Increased responsibilities for patient management and for patient referrals increase their value under managed care. To date, however, the financial incentives for physicians have been for greater specialization. Medical school faculty encourage specialization, specialists are considered more prestigious, they earn much higher incomes than primary care physicians, and, considering the size of their educational debt when they graduate, a specialist is more likely to be able to repay it in a shorter time period. New medical graduates are four times more likely to choose a career in high-technology specialties such as cardiology, gastroenterology, and orthopedics than in primary care. As managed care systems rely on fewer specialists, their incomes will decline. This is beginning to occur in more competitive markets for physician services, such as in California, where they are not as busy as they once were.

The Medicare system, which pays for almost 30 percent of total physician expenditures, is still primarily a fee-for-service system without gatekeepers to decrease the use of specialists. Even though the new Medicare relative value payment system has lowered procedure-oriented specialists' fees, specialists are still well paid relative to physicians who provide cognitive and patient management services (Pope and Schneider 1992). Until the Medicare system relies more on managed care or dramatically lowers specialists' fees, specialists who serve large numbers of Medicare patients will have higher incomes than those who are more dependent upon private patients in competitive managed care markets, such as in California. The excess capacity that exists among specialists will eventually decrease the disparity in specialist incomes between those working in different regions of the United States and serving different portions of Medicare and managed care patients.

The trend in the physician services market is for an increased decision-making role for the primary care physician, as he or she determine referral patterns in a competitive system based on managed care. The consequence of this new competitive environment will be declining specialty services (and incomes) for specialists and an increased role (and incomes) for primary care physicians.

Note

1. Physician incomes are highly skewed; that is, the physician income distribution contains large values at the high end of the income distribution. Therefore using the average income per physician is a less accurate measure of the "typical" physician's income. It is for this reason that the middle of the income distribution, the median, is used.

Reference

Pope, G. C., and J. E. Schneider. "Trends in Physician Income." *Health Affairs* 11 (Spring 1992): 181–93.

11

The Malpractice Crisis

History of the Malpractice Crisis

Malpractice entered a "crisis" in the early 1970s when physicians' malpractice premiums rose from $6,628 in 1974 to $10,828 in 1976, and for some specialties, such as obstetrics/gynecology and surgery, the increases were even greater (see Figure 11.1). During this first "malpractice crisis," some insurers completely withdrew from the malpractice insurance market, while others increased their premiums by as much as 300 percent. Physicians threatened to strike if state legislatures did not intervene. To ensure access to malpractice insurance at the lowest possible rates, some medical societies formed their own insurance companies. By the late 1970s and early 1980s, malpractice premiums had stabilized somewhat, but they rose sharply again in the mid-1980s, precipitating another "malpractice crisis." Again, physicians demanded that state legislators do something.

By the late 1980s, malpractice premiums and awards had again stabilized, and claims filed against physicians declined, from an average of 10.2 per 100 physicians in 1985 to 7.7 in 1990, as shown in Figure 11.2. For obstetricians, who have the highest number of claims filed, the drop was greater, from 25.8 to 11.9. Malpractice premiums as a percent of total physician expenses rose from 7.4 percent in 1982 to a high of 12.1 percent in 1987 and then declined to 9.0 percent in 1991 (see Figure 11.3). For obstetricians and anesthesiologists, premiums declined from 20 and 30 percent in 1987, to 16 and 23 percent, respectively, in 1990.

Figure 11.1   Medical Professional Liability Insurance Premiums for
Self-Employed Physicians, 1974–1991

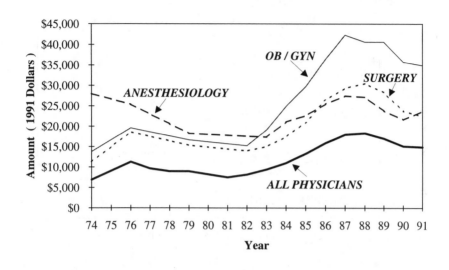

Source: American Medical Association (Chicago, IL), *Socioeconomic Characteristics of Medical Practice*, various editions.

An interesting aspect of the rising costs for malpractice insurance is the difference between the average (mean) jury award and the median jury award, which represents the midpoint of all the awards (one-half the awards are above and one-half below the median award), both of which have risen over time (see Figure 11.4). In 1990, the average jury award ($1,763,876) was much greater than the median award ($450,000), meaning there are many small awards and few large ones, though the latter receive the greatest publicity.

The current respite in the malpractice crisis is probably temporary; most likely, as shown in Figure 11.5, the cycle will repeat itself, and there will be further calls for legislative action.

It is not clear why these crises recur. Two reasons for the increase in malpractice cases are, first, physicians are performing more procedures, using complex new technologies, which carry greater risks of injury. Second, liberalized applications of tort law have created uncertainty among insurers concerning awards for "pain and suffering" and have placed some defendants ("deep pockets") at greater financial risk, even though

Figure 11.2   Average Incidence of Medical Professional Liability
Claims by Specialty, 1985–1991

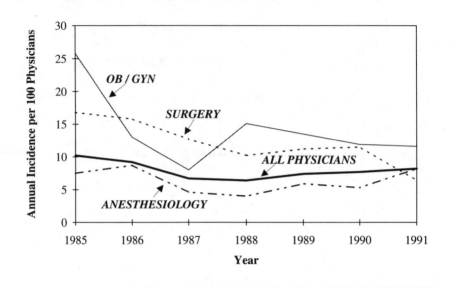

Source: American Medical Association (Chicago, IL), *Socioeconomic Characteristics of Medical Practice*, various editions.

their contributions to injuries may be minor. (The United States is also a litigious society.) It is clear, however, that rising malpractice premiums are *not* due to collusion among insurers. There are a large number of insurers, including physician-owned insurance companies (although there are fewer companies from whom these insurance companies purchase reinsurance), and there is a great deal of competition among them.

Objectives of the Malpractice System

Tort law is the basis for medical malpractice. It entitles an injured person compensation as a result of someone's negligence. Damages include economic losses (lost wages and medical bills) and "pain and suffering." Thus physicians have a financial incentive to provide good treatment and to perform only those procedures for which they are competent. The two purposes of tort law are compensation to the victim for negligence and deterrence of future negligence.

How well does the malpractice system fulfill these two objectives?

Figure 11.3   Malpractice Premiums as a Percentage of Total
Physician Expenses, 1982–1991

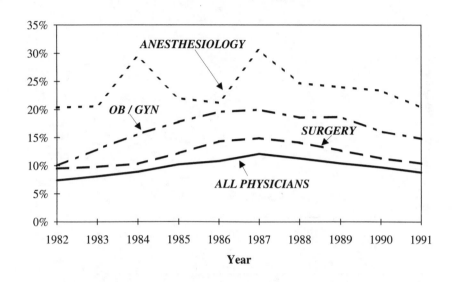

Sources: American Medical Association (Chicago, IL), *The Profile of Medical Practice* and *Socioeconomic Characteristics of Physicians,* various editions.

Can legislative reforms achieve these objectives at lower cost than the current system? Physician advocates maintain that too many claims are filed that have little to do with negligence (so the insurer will settle to avoid legal expense), and that juries award large sums that are unrelated to actual damages. Further, "defensive" medicine—additional tests prescribed by physicians to protect themselves against malpractice claims—add billions of dollars to the nation's health expenditures.

Patient advocates claim there is more extensive physician negligence than is reflected by the number of claims filed, that large jury awards are infrequent, that incompetent physicians must be discouraged from practicing because physicians do not adequately monitor themselves, and that defensive medicine is caused by an insurance system that eliminates patients' incentives to be concerned about the cost of care.

Compensation of Victims

Which arguments are correct? A 1990 Harvard University study found that too few of those injured by negligence are compensated under the

Figure 11.4   Jury Awards for Medical Professional Liability Cases, 1974–1990

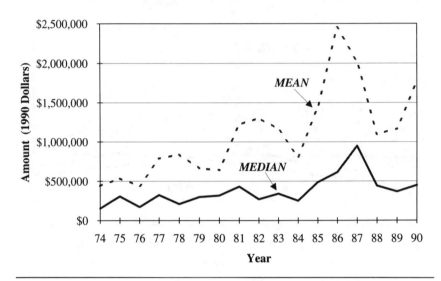

Source: American College of Surgeons (Chicago, IL), *Socioeconomic Factbook*, various editions.

malpractice system (Localio et al. 1991). The authors examined hospital records in 51 New York hospitals and determined that almost 4 percent of all patients suffered an injury while in the hospital and that one-quarter of those injuries were the result of negligence. Thus about 1 percent of all hospital discharges in New York in 1984 were due to negligence. Examples of injuries occurring in hospitals are errors in diagnosis, falls, hospital-caused infections, and surgical complications.

Surprisingly, less than 2 percent of the patients identified as victims of negligence filed a malpractice claim. Six percent of injured patients who had not been victims of negligence also filed claims. According to the Harvard researchers, only one-half of patient claims filed eventually received some compensation. Most settle within two years without receiving any compensation, and the rest may wait years. Few negligence victims ever receive compensation. About 1 percent of malpractice victims receive some compensation. Of those patients injured through negligence and who do not file claims (98 percent of negligence victims), 20 percent of those negligent injuries were serious—disabilities that lasted 6 months or more, including fatalities.

Physicians, 1975–1991

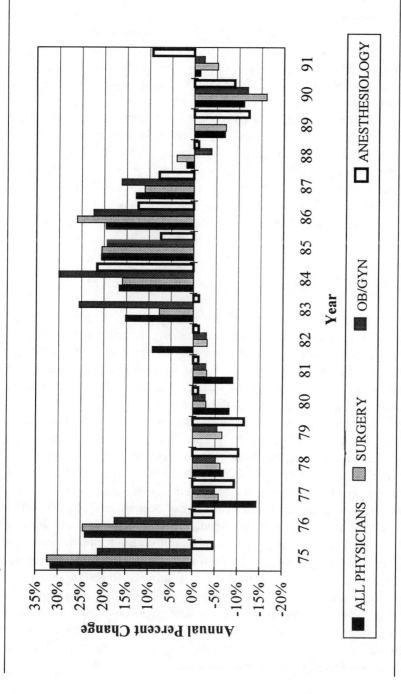

Sources: American Medical Association (Chicago, IL), *The Profile of Medical Practice* and *Socioeconomic Characteristics of Medical Practice,* various editions.

Several reasons account for the low percentage of negligence claims filed: A patient may not know that negligence caused an injury. Some claims may be difficult to prove. Recoverable damages may be less than the litigation costs, particularly when the injured patient earns low wages, which explains the low incidence of claims for minor injuries.

The cost of administering the compensation system are very high, and only a small portion of malpractice premiums, 28–40 percent, are returned to those injured through negligence. Overhead, including legal fees, consumes the major portion of premiums. Health insurance, on the other hand, returns 90 percent of the premium for medical expenses.

If the sole purpose of malpractice insurance were to compensate those negligently injured, more efficient ways are available, at lower administrative costs. A different approach could compensate a greater number of victims and return a greater portion of premiums to those injured.

Deterrence of Negligence

Justification of the current malpractice system must depend, then, on how well it performs its second, more important, role—the prevention of negligence. Compensation tries not only to make whole the damages suffered by the victims of negligence but to have negligent health care providers pay that compensation so they will exercise greater caution in future care-giving situations. There is increasing concern, however, that not enough injuries are prevented (deterrence effect) by the current system to justify the high costs of practicing defensive medicine to prevent claims, determining fault, and prosecuting malpractice claims.

The standard of care used in determining negligence is what one would expect from a reasonably competent person, exercising care, and knowledgeable about advances in medicine. Some cases of malpractice are easily established, such as amputating the wrong leg and leaving surgical supplies in a patient's abdomen. With other forms of physician behavior, however, there are uncertainties in both diagnosis and in the outcome of medical treatment. Many medical procedures are inherently risky. Even with correct diagnosis and treatment, a patient may die because of poor health conditions. A baby may be born with a birth defect through no fault of the obstetrician. It is true that physicians differ in the quality of care they provide and in their success rates, but it is difficult, hence costly, to determine whether a specific outcome is a result of physician negligence, poor communication of the risks involved, or due to the patient's underlying health condition.

The potential for malpractice suits increases the cost to the physician of negligent behavior. Physicians would therefore be expected to change their behavior and restrict their practice to forestall such costs. They would no longer perform procedures and tasks for which they lack competence. The deterrence effect should cause physicians to exercise proper care to minimize errors. Prevention costs time and resources; therefore physicians should invest in prevention (their time, training, and medical testing) up to the point where the additional cost of prevention equals the additional value of injuries avoided (foregone malpractice costs). "Too much" prevention could occur if a great deal of time and resources (the additional costs) are used for preventing occasional minor injuries. A requirement that the injury rate be zero would be too costly for society. It would mean that skilled specialists would be discouraged from performing procedures that involve an element of risk of injury but from which the patient could benefit.

How well does the malpractice system deter negligence? More precisely, is the value (to patients) of the negligence prevented greater than the costs (defensive medicine, determining liability, and litigation) of the malpractice system? Experts differ on this issue.

Critics of the current system claim that physicians are not penalized by negligence, since only 2 percent of negligence victims filed claims, as described in the study on negligence in New York hospitals. Second, since less than one-half of malpractice insurance premiums, which are approximately $9 billion, or 1 percent of total health care spending, are returned to victims of negligence and the remainder is spent on overhead and legal fees, the malpractice system is too costly. Third, since most malpractice insurance does not "experience rate" physicians within their specialty, incompetent physicians are not penalized by higher premiums; their behavior merely increases premiums for all physicians in that specialty. Fourth, not all physicians who are sued are incompetent. Although incompetent physicians may be sued more often, other physicians are also sued because of occasional errors or because they are specialists who treat more difficult cases; board-certified physicians are sued more often than other physicians.

Lastly, the current system results in high costs for tests and services not medically justified but performed to protect physicians from malpractice claims (defensive medicine). Physicians overuse tests because the costs of such defensive medicine are borne by patients and insurers, while an injury claim could result in physician liability. Thus physicians are able to shift the costs of their exercising greater caution to others.

Defenders of the malpractice system claim that the incentive to avoid malpractice suits changes physician behavior and makes them act more carefully. Physicians have limited their scope of practice, they are more conscientious in documenting their records, and they take the time to discuss the risks involved in a procedure with their patients. Even though premiums of physicians are not experience-rated, lawsuits are a costly deterrent in terms of time spent defending themselves and potential loss of reputation.

The costs of defensive medicine are probably overstated, since excessive testing would remain even if the threat of malpractice were eliminated. Physicians order too many tests because insured patients pay only a small portion of the price for physician-ordered tests. Even though the benefits to the patient of the tests are less than the costs of performing those tests, it is rational for patients to want those tests because their benefits may be greater than their share of the costs. Physicians reimbursed fee-for-service also benefit by prescribing extra tests. Physicians in HMOs have less of an incentive to perform excessive testing. Thus physicans' use of excessive testing results, in part, from traditional insurance payment systems and a lack of policing of such tests by insurers, not necessarily from malpractice.

A recent study that estimated the cost of defensive medicine concluded that it is very difficult to determine the additional costs solely attributable to fear of malpractice claims. The authors did, however, estimate the costs of defensive medicine at $4 billion in 1994 and $36 billion over the period 1994–1998, a very small percent of total medical expenditures (Rubin and Mendelson 1993).

Further, removing the threat of malpractice leaves few alternatives for monitoring and disciplining physicians. The emphasis by organized medicine on quality control has always been on the "process" of becoming a physician, that is, the number of years of education, graduation from an approved medical school, and passing national examinations. However, once a physician is licensed, he or she is never reexamined for relicensure. State medical licensing boards do not adequately monitor physician quality nor discipline incompetent physicians. Lastly, patients have little or no access to information on physicians' procedure outcomes. Until recently, the medical profession actively discouraged public access to such information. What recourse, other than filing a malpractice claim, would a patient have after being injured by an incompetent physician?

Victims of negligence are not adequately compensated—there is little disagreement on that. The controversial issues are whether malpractice actually deters negligence and whether alternatives are available for monitoring and disciplining incompetent physician behavior.

Proposed Changes to the Malpractice System

Many changes have been proposed to correct perceived inadequacies of the malpractice system. Proposals to limit the potential recovery of damages have the effect of decreasing the value of malpractice claims and thereby reduce the number of malpractice claims filed. For example, limiting damages for "pain and suffering" would reduce the amount of malpractice awards that can be used to pay legal fees, since the remainder of the award is for lost wages and medical expenses. Reducing awards by amounts already paid to the victim by other sources, such as health insurers, would have the same effect. Lawyers will have a lessened incentive to bring suits on behalf of patients. Similarly, fewer cases would be brought if a limit were placed on lawyers' contingency fees (currently these can be as high as one-third to one-half of the award). Lawyers would have less incentive to invest their resources on cases whose awards would be smaller. Lawyers are in a competitive market and may represent either plaintiffs or defendants in malpractice cases. Lawyers for defendants are paid hourly rates. Fewer lawyers would choose to represent plaintiffs if contingency fees were reduced.

Proposals that make it more difficult to prove a malpractice claim, such as using local rather than national standards and excluding testimony from out-of-state experts, reduce the number of claims by reducing the cases to which lawyers would be willing to devote their own time and resources.

Proposals that lessen the size of an award or that make it more difficult to bring claims are addressing the wrong problem. These "remedies" are directed at decreasing the number of claims, while the real problem appears to be that too few negligent claims are brought. Malpractice reforms should be evaluated in terms of whether they deter negligent behavior and improve victim compensation.

No-Fault Malpractice

One proposed reform, a "no fault" system, would compensate an injured patient, whether or not negligence was involved. In return, patients would forfeit their right to sue. The main advantages of a no-fault system are, first, litigation costs would be lower since it would not be necessary to prove who was at fault for the injury and these savings could be used to increase victim compensation; second, all injured patients would receive some compensation, most of whom could not win malpractice suits because their claims were either too small to attract a lawyer's interest or because no one was at fault in causing their injury. A no-fault system could have a schedule of payments, according to types of injuries, to compensate the injured for loss of income and for medical expenses. In cases of severe injury, the schedule could include payment for "pain and suffering."

A no-fault system has, however, two important problems. First, under such a system, there is no deterrence mechanism to weed out incompetent providers or to encourage physicians to exercise greater caution. Second, because all injuries would be compensable, no clear line is drawn between injuries that result from negligence, injuries that are not the result of negligence, unfavorable treatment outcomes because of the patient's health condition and lifestyle, and outcomes of risky procedures that are never 100 percent favorable, such as transplant procedures and future health problems of low-birthweight infants. Compensating patients for all injuries and unfavorable outcomes could be very expensive, given the large number of injuries cited earlier in the Harvard study for which no claims were filed. And who should bear these costs?

Methods for deterring physician negligence continue to be difficult to resolve. Regulatory approaches, such as state licensing boards for monitoring and disciplining physicians, have performed poorly. Until other deterrent mechanisms are in place, it would be premature to eliminate the malpractice system.

Enterprise Liability

One approach that seeks to improve upon the malpractice system for deterring negligence is referred to as "enterprise liability." Changing the liability laws so that liability is shifted away from the physician (they can no longer be sued) to a larger entity of which the physician is a part, such as a hospital, medical group, or managed care organization, would place the incentive for monitoring and enforcing medical quality on that larger organization. These organizations would balance the increased costs of prevention and risk-reducing behavior versus the potential for a malpractice claim.

The shift to enterprise liability is already occurring because of market trends and court rulings. The growth of managed care organizations and the fact that they are liable for those physicians whom they employ or contract with has increased such organizations' monitoring of physician behavior. Further, the concept of "joint and several" liability, wherein the physician is the primary defendant but the hospital or HMO is also named as a defendant with potentially 100 percent liability for damages (even though they may have been only 10 percent at fault), provides hospitals and HMOs with an incentive to increase their quality assurance and risk management programs. Many physicians, however, perform surgery only in outpatient settings, do not practice within a hospital, and do not belong to large health plans. These physicians would be most affected by such a shift in liability laws since they would lose some of their autonomy as they become subject to greater supervision by larger entities.

Placing liability for malpractice on a larger organization would enable insurers to experience-rate the organization. As more health care organizations become experience-rated, they will devote more resources to monitoring the quality of care and the disciplining of physicians for poor performance. Many organizations, such as HMOs, PPOs, and large medical groups, have information systems in place to profile the practice patterns of their physicians. Competition among health care organizations over price and quality provides them with an incentive to develop quality control mechanisms. These organizations, rather than regulatory bodies, have both the incentives and the ability to evaluate and control physicians.

Summary

Experts do not agree on malpractice reform (see, for example, the proposals of Newhouse and Weiler 1991 and Danzon 1991). Victim compensation could be improved under a no-fault system, but incentives for deterring negligence would be lacking. Proposals for change often reflect the interests of those who might benefit. Medical societies are often pitted against the trial lawyers' association. The battle for changes in the malpractice system are occurring in almost every state, and there is talk of federal legislation. All proposals for reform, by whatever interest group, should be judged by how well they achieve the two goals of the malpractice system: compensation for victims injured by negligence and deterrence of future negligence.

References

Danzon, P. M. "Liability for Medical Malpractice." *Journal of Economic Perspectives* 5 (Summer 1991): 51–69.

Localio, A. R., A. G. Lawthers, T. A. Brennan, N. M. Laird, L. E. Hebert, L. M. Peterson, J. P. Newhouse, P. C. Weiler, and H. H. Hiatt. "Relation between Malpractice Claims and Adverse Events Due to Negligence." *New England Journal of Medicine* 325 (25 July 1991): 245–51.

Newhouse, J. P., and P. C. Weiler. "Reforming Medical Malpractice and Insurance." *Regulation* 14 (Fall 1991): 78–84.

Rubin, R. J., and D. Mendelson, *Estimating the Costs of Defensive Medicine.* Fairfax, Virginia: Lewin-VHI, Inc., 1993.

12

Competition among Hospitals: Does It Raise or Lower Costs?

Current federal policy (the antitrust laws) encourages competition among hospitals. Hospitals proposing a merger are scrutinized by the Federal Trade Commission (FTC) to determine whether the merger will lessen hospital competition in that market, in which case the FTC will oppose the merger. Critics of this policy believe that hospitals should be permitted, in fact encouraged, to consolidate and cooperate in the facilities and services that they provide. They claim that the result will be greater efficiencies, less duplication of costly services, and higher quality of care. Who is correct and what is appropriate public policy for hospitals—competition or cooperation?

Important to understanding hospital performance are, first, the methods used to pay hospitals (different payment methods provide hospitals with different incentives) and, second, the consequences of having different numbers of hospitals compete with one another.

The Origins of Nonprice Competition

After the introduction of Medicare and Medicaid in 1966, hospitals were paid their costs for the services they rendered to the aged and poor. Private insurance, which was widespread among the remainder of the population, also reimbursed hospitals generously, either according to their costs or their charges. The extensive coverage of hospital services by both private and public payers removed patients' incentives to be concerned

119

with the costs of hospital care. Patients pay less out-of-pocket for hospital care (10 percent) than for any other medical service.

There were virtually no incentives on the part of third party payers (government and private insurance) and patients to be concerned with hospital efficiency and duplication of facilities and services. Further, most hospitals are organized as not-for-profit (nongovernment) organizations either affiliated with a religious organization or controlled by boards of trustees selected from the community. With the introduction of extensive public and private hospital insurance after the mid-1960s, the use of non-profit hospitals increased. Lacking a profit motive and being assured of their survival by the generous payment methods, nonprofit hospitals also had no incentive to be concerned with efficiency. The effect of the lack of efficiency incentives was that the costs of caring for patients rose rapidly.

Figure 12.1 illustrates the dramatic rise in hospital expenditures from the 1960s to the present. After Medicare and Medicaid were en-acted in 1965, hospital expenditures increased by more than 16 percent per year. These large increases were primarily due to sharp increases in hospital prices, as shown in Figure 12.2. Hospital price increases moderated during the early 1970s when wage and price controls were imposed, but then increased sharply once they were removed in mid-1974. Hospital expenditure increases were less rapid in the mid- to late 1980s as DRGs were implemented and price competition increased.[1]

In the late 1960s the private sector also did not encourage efficiency. Services that could be provided less expensively in an outpatient setting (such as diagnostic workups) were only reimbursed by Blue Cross if the patient stayed overnight in the hospital. Small hospitals attempted to emulate medical centers by having the latest in technology, even though those services were infrequently used. It did not matter whether larger organizations had lower costs per unit and higher-quality outcomes than smaller facilities because cost was of little concern to patients or to the purchasers of the service.

The greater the number of hospitals in a community, the more intense was the competition among the nonprofit hospitals to become the most prestigious hospital. Hospitals competed for physicians by offering the physicians all the services available at other hospitals so that the physician's productivity and convenience of caring for patients would be increased and so that the physician would not have to refer their patient to another hospital. This form of nonprice competition was characterized as a "medical arms race" and was wasteful and resulted in rapidly rising hospital expenditures.

Figure 12.1 Trends in Hospital Expenditures, 1966–1991

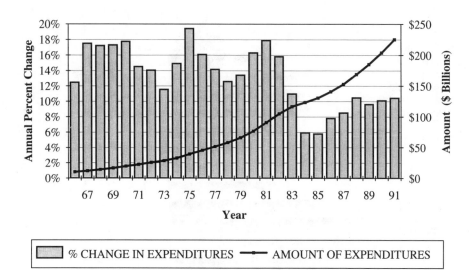

Note: Figures are for nonfederal short-term general (STG) hospitals.
Source: American Hospital Association (Chicago, IL), *Hospital Statistics, 1990–1991.*

As the costs of nonprice competition increased, the federal and state governments attempted to change hospitals' behavior. Regulations were enacted to control hospital capital expenditures; hospitals were required to have certificate-of-need (CON) approval from a state planning agency before they could undertake large investments. According to proponents of state planning, controlling hospital investment would eliminate unnecessary and duplicative investments. Unfortunately, no attempts were made to change hospital payment methods, which would have changed hospitals' incentives to undertake such investments.

Numerous studies concluded that CON did not have any effect on limiting the growth in hospital investment. Instead, CON was used in an anticompetitive manner to benefit existing hospitals in the community, who ended up controlling the CON approval process. Ambulatory surgicenters (unaffiliated with hospitals) could not receive CON approval for construction because they would take away hospital patients; health maintenance organizations, such as Kaiser, found it difficult to enter a new market because they could not receive CON approval to build a

Figure 12.2 Annual Percent Changes in the Consumer Price Index and the Hospital Room Price Index, 1965–1992

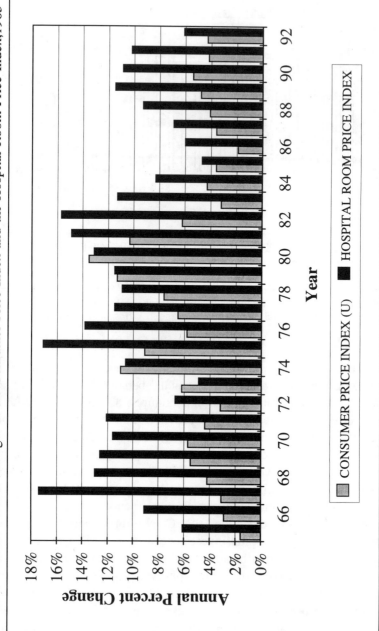

Note: CPI (U) = consumer price index for all urban consumers.

Sources: U.S. Bureau of the Census (Washington, DC), *Statistical Abstract of the United States and Historical Abstract of the United States,* various editions.

new hospital; and the courts found that the CON process was used in an "arbitrary and capricious manner" against for-profit hospitals attempting to enter the market of an existing nonprofit hospital.

The Transition to Price Competition

Until the 1980s, hospital competition was synonymous with nonprice competition and its effect was unnecessary and rapidly rising expenditures (Robinson and Luft 1987).

During the 1980s hospitals' and purchasers' incentives changed. Medicare began to pay hospitals a fixed price per admission (which varied according to the type of admission). This new payment system, referred to as diagnostic-related groups (DRGs), was phased in over five years, starting in 1983. Faced with a fixed price, hospitals now had an incentive to reduce their costs of caring for aged patients. In addition to becoming more efficient, lengths of stay for aged patients were reduced, which caused declines in hospital occupancy rates. And, for the first time, hospitals became concerned with their physicians' practice behaviors. If physicians ordered too many tests or kept the patient longer than necessary in the hospital, then, given the fixed DRG price, the hospital lost money.

As employers became concerned over their employees' rising medical expenses, they pressured their insurers to reduce the cost of the largest and fastest-growing component of medical expenditures—hospital services. The result was that insurers changed their insurance benefits to encourage patients to have diagnostic tests and minor surgical procedures performed in an outpatient setting. Insurers instituted utilization review to monitor the appropriateness of inpatient admissions, and this further reduced hospital admissions and lengths of stay. The effect of these changes in hospital and purchaser incentives was a further reduction in hospital occupancy rates, from 76 percent in 1980 to 65 percent by 1985, where it has since remained. The decline in occupancy rates was much more severe for small hospitals, going below 50 percent.

As hospital occupancy rates declined, hospitals were willing to negotiate price discounts with those insurers and HMOs able to deliver a large number of patients to their hospitals. The result was that by the late 1980s price competition started among hospitals.

Price competition does not imply that hospitals compete only on the basis of which hospital has the lowest price. Purchasers are also interested in other characteristics of that hospital, such as what facilities and services are available, how close the hospital is to their patient population, patient satisfaction, and treatment outcomes.

Price Competition in Theory

How likely are hospitals to respond to this new competitive environment where purchasers demand lower prices, high patient satisfaction, and information on hospital outcomes? Let us examine two hypothetical situations. The first is where there is only one hospital in an area. Being the only hospital, there are no competitors and no substitutes for inpatient services; the hospital is a monopolist in the provision of hospital services. As a monopolist, the hospital has no incentive to respond to purchaser demands for lower prices, quality information, and patient satisfaction. The purchaser has no choice but to use the only hospital available. If the hospital is not efficient, it can pass those higher costs on to the purchaser. If the patients are dissatisfied with the hospital's services or the hospital refuses to provide outcomes information on its open-heart surgery facility, the purchaser and patients have no choice but to use the only hospital in town. (Obviously, at some point it becomes worthwhile for patients to incur large travel costs to go to distant hospitals or for the purchaser to induce another hospital to enter the market.)

When only one hospital serves a market, that hospital is unlikely to have good performance. The hospital has little incentive to be efficient or to respond to purchaser and patient demands.

The second hypothetical scenario consists of many hospitals, perhaps ten, serving a particular geographic area. Now let us assume that there is a large employer in the area who is interested in lowering its employees' hospital costs and is also interested in the quality and satisfaction of the care received, and, for simplicity, that each of the ten hospitals are equally accessible to the firm's employees (both with regard to distance and staff appointments for the employees' physicians). How are hospitals likely to respond to this employer's demands?

At least several of the hospitals would be willing, in return for receiving a large number of patients from that employer, to negotiate lower prices and accede to the employer's demands for information on quality and patient satisfaction. As long as the price the hospital receives from that employer is greater than the direct costs of caring for their patients, the hospital will make more money than if it did not accept those patients. Further, unless the hospitals in that market were as efficient as the others, they could not hope to win such contracts. A more efficient hospital would always be able to underprice them.

Similar to competing on price is the competition that would occur among hospitals on willingness to provide information on treatment outcomes. As long as the hospitals have to rely on purchaser revenues to survive, they will be driven to respond to purchaser demands. Unless they are responsive to purchaser demands, other hospitals would be and they would soon find that they have too few patients to remain in business.

When hospitals compete on price, quality, and on other purchaser requirements, their performance is opposite that of a monopoly provider of hospital services. Hospitals have an incentive to be efficient and to respond to purchaser demands in price-competitive markets.

What if, instead of competing with each other, the ten hospitals decided to agree among themselves not to compete on price nor provide purchasers with any additional information? The outcome would be similar to a monopoly situation. Prices would be higher, and hospitals would have less incentive to be efficient. Patients would be worse off since they would pay more for their hospital care, and patient quality and patient satisfaction would be lower since employers and other purchasers would be unable to select hospitals based on patient quality and satisfaction information.

The antitrust laws are designed to prevent hospitals from acting anticompetitively. Price-fixing agreements, such as described above, are illegal because they lessen competition among hospitals. Barriers that prevent competitors from entering a market are also anticompetitive. If two hospitals in a market are able to restrict entry into that market (perhaps through the use of regulations such as CON), they will have greater monopoly power, and they will be less price competitive and less responsive to purchaser demands. Mergers may be similarly anticompetitive. For example, if the ten hospitals merged so that only two hospital organizations remained, the degree of competition would be less than when there were ten such competitors. It is for this reason that the FTC examines hospital mergers to determine whether they will lessen competition in the market.

Price Competition in Practice

The above discussion provides a theoretical basis for price competition. To move from its theoretical benefits to reality, it is necessary to consider two questions: First, are there enough hospitals in any market for price competition to occur? Second, is there any evidence on the actual effects of hospital price competition?

The number of competing hospitals in a market is determined by the cost-size relationship of hospitals (economies of scale) and the size of the market (the population served). A larger-sized hospital, for example 200 beds, is likely to have lower average costs per patient than a hospital that has only 50 beds with the same set of services because in a larger hospital some costs can be spread over a greater number of patients. For example, some costs will be the same regardless of whether there are 50 or 200 patients, such as an administrator, an x-ray technician, and x-ray equipment, which can be used more fully in a larger organization. These economies of scale (size), however, do not continue indefinitely; at some point the higher costs of coordination of services begin to exceed the gains accruing from a larger size. Studies have generally indicated that hospitals in the size range of 200–400 beds have the lowest average cost.

If the population in an area consists of only 100,000, then only one hospital of 260 beds is likely to survive (assuming 800 patient days per thousand and an 80 percent occupancy). If there were more than one hospital, each would have higher average costs than one larger hospital; one of the hospitals would expand, achieve lower average costs, and be able to underprice the other hospital. An area with a population of 1,000,000 is large enough to support between three and six hospitals.

Hospital services, however, are not all the same. The economies of scale associated with an obstetrics facility are quite different than those associated with organ transplant services. Patients are also less willing to travel large distances for a normal delivery than for a heart transplant; the travel costs of going to another state for a transplant represent a smaller portion of the total cost of the service (and the travel time is less crucial) than for giving birth. Thus the number of competitors in a market depends upon the particular service; for some services the relevant geographic market served may be relatively small, while for others it may be the state or region.

Approximately 80 percent of hospital beds are located in metropolitan statistical areas (MSAs). While an MSA may not necessarily be indicative of the particular market in which a hospital competes, since for some services the travel time within an MSA may be too great while for others the market may encompass multiple MSAs, the number of hospitals within an MSA provides a general indication of the number of competitors within a hospital's market. As shown in Figure 12.3, 160 MSAs (or 43 percent) have less than four hospitals and 76 MSAs (24 percent) have four or five hospitals. The remaining MSAs (33 percent) have more than six hospitals. However, these 33 percent of MSAs with six or more hospitals contain 80 percent of the hospitals located in metropolitan areas. Thus the large majority of hospitals in MSAs (80 percent) are located in MSAs with six or more hospitals. Even within an MSA with few hospitals, substitutes are often available to the hospitals' service, for example, outpatient surgery, which decreases those hospitals' monopoly power.

When there are few providers of specialized facilities in a market (because of economies of scale and the size of the market), the relevant geographic market is likely to be much larger because the demand for highly specialized services is generally not of an emergency nature and patients are more willing to travel. Several insurers negotiate prices for transplants with several regional Centers of Excellence, hospitals who perform a high number of transplants and have good outcomes.

Figure 12.3   The Number of Hospitals in Metropolitan Statistical Areas, 1991

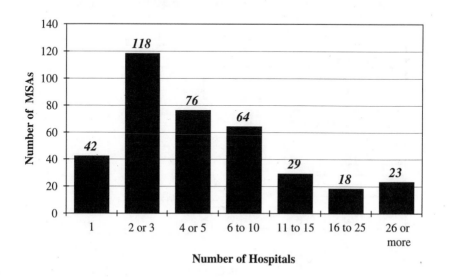

Source: American Hospital Association (Chicago, IL), *Hospital Statistics, 1992–1993*, Table 6.

It would thus appear that price competition among hospitals is feasible. As insurers and large employers have become concerned over the costs of hospital care and are becoming better informed on hospital prices and patient outcomes, hospitals are being forced to be responsive to purchaser demands and compete according to price, outcomes, and patient satisfaction.

Recent studies on hospital price competition support traditional economic expectations regarding competitive hospital markets. Compared to the rest of the United States and to states that regulate hospital rates (such as Maryland, New York, New Jersey, and Massachusetts), California, which has had a much more competitive environment in the 1980s, has had a much lower rate of increase in hospital expenses per capita (see Figure 12.4).

Within California, Melnick and Zwanziger (1988) classified hospitals according to the competitiveness of their markets. They found that hospitals in more-competitive markets in the mid-1980s had a lower rate of increase in their costs per discharge and cost per capita than did hospitals in less-competitive markets.

Figure 12.4   Comparison of Inflation-Adjusted Cumulative Growth in Per Capita Hospital Expenditures, 1980–1991

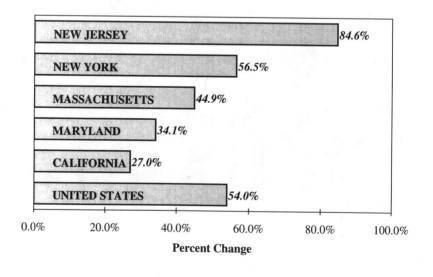

Source: Calculations of Professor Glenn Melnick, UCLA-RAND Corporation.

Lower hospital costs were also passed on to purchasers in the form of lower prices. In a subsequent study using data on prices actually paid for hospital care by a large insurer, Melnick et al. (1992) found that California Blue Cross was able to receive greater price discounts from hospitals located in more-competitive markets. The researchers also found that hospitals with high occupancy rates charged much higher prices. These findings imply that hospital mergers that decrease competition and reduce excess capacity are therefore likely to result in higher hospital prices.

Summary

The controversy over whether hospital competition results in higher or lower costs is based on studies from two different time periods. When hospitals were paid according to their costs, nonprice competition occurred and resulted in rapidly rising hospital costs. The change in hospital payment according to fixed prices by Medicare and negotiated prices by private payers changed hospitals' incentives. Hospitals now have incentives to be efficient and to compete on price with private payers. The consequence is that hospital costs and prices have risen less rapidly in more-competitive hospital markets. Public policy, such as the antitrust laws, that encourage competitive hospital markets will be of greater benefit to purchasers and patients than policies that enable hospitals to increase their monopoly power.

Note

1. A recent study has shown that starting in the mid-1980s hospital price increases have been greatly overstated since they measure "list" prices rather than actual prices charged. The difference between the two has become greater with the increase in hospital discounting (Dranove, Shanley, and White 1991).

References

Dranove, D., M. Shanley, and W. White. "How Fast Are Hospital Prices Really Rising?" *Medical Care* 29 (August 1991): 690–96.

Melnick, G. A., J. Zwanziger, A. Bamezai, and R. Pattison. "The Effects of Market Structure and Bargaining Position on Hospital Prices." *Journal of Health Economics* 11 (1992): 217–33.

Melnick, G. A., and J. Zwanziger. "Hospital Behavior under Competition and Cost Containment Policies." *Journal of the American Medical Association* 260 (8 November 1988): 2669–75.

Robinson, J., and H. Luft. "Competition and the Cost of Hospital Care, 1972–1982." *Journal of the American Medical Association* 257 (19 June 1987): 3241–45.

13

Vertically Integrated
Health Care Organizations

Health care organizations are changing. Twenty-five years ago the typical medical delivery system in this country consisted of a not-for-profit hospital and its medical staff, who were in either solo or small group practice. Diagnostic workups and surgical procedures were predominately performed in the hospital, and the home was not considered to be a setting where the patient could be cared for. Insurers, such as Blue Cross, were strictly payers of hospital services.

Today, both the settings where health care is delivered and the functions performed by different organizations have changed. Insurers have developed their own medical delivery systems; hospitals are affiliated with other hospitals, they may market directly to employers, some even own physicians' practices, and some hospitals have formed their own HMOs.

Why have these changes occurred and what is the health care organization of tomorrow likely to look like?

Each organizational structure offers certain benefits but also contains some offsetting disadvantages (costs). The organizational form that will grow and become predominant will be one whose benefits clearly outweigh its costs. Similarly, the reason organizational structures change is because there has been a change in the benefits or the costs of certain types of organizations, making them either more or less desirable.

Two important trends have caused health care organizations to change: The first, and most important, is changes in payment for medical services; the second is medical technology.

Independent Hospitals and Physicians

Until the early 1980s, hospitals and physicians were separately reimbursed fee-for-service for the services they provided. Patients, who had
extensive insurance for hospital and in-hospital physician services, had
little concern with the costs of their care. Hospitals and physicians'
offices were the only settings in which care was provided and reimbursed
by insurers, such as Blue Cross and Blue Shield. Neither the hospital
nor physician was financially affected (or in any way at risk) by the
payment the other provider received. Further, the hospital was paid
according to its costs of providing that care, regardless of how high
those costs were. Hospitals were independent from other hospitals and
physicians practiced by themselves or in small groups. This organizational form, which provided maximum autonomy to the hospital and to
the medical staff, offered the providers the greatest benefits relative to
their costs.

Economic efficiency, which was low, was not a concern to either
the physicians or to the hospital. Hospitals were paid their costs, and
they engaged in nonprice competition, namely, investing in facilities and
services, such as open-heart surgery units, which were little used but
made the institution more prestigious.

The Move toward Horizontal Integration

The first major change in organizational form, horizontal integration, began in the 1970s when hospitals began to affiliate and form multihospital
systems. The stimulus for this change was a concern by some insurers
with the rising costs of hospital care. As hospital efficiency increased
in importance, hospitals sought to take advantage of economies of scale,
that is, the lower (average) costs associated with larger volume. Hospitals
participated in joint purchasing arrangements with other hospitals, which
enabled each hospital to receive a larger discount on its supply purchases.
These hospital relationships offered some benefits (lower production
costs) at very little loss in autonomy.

As efficiency became more important to some hospitals, stronger
affiliations formed. Hospitals became part of larger hospital systems.
The economies derived from these relationships were greater: a larger
organization could receive lower interest rates on its bond financings, the
costs of specialized hospital personnel (such as reimbursement specialists) could be spread among more hospitals, and construction costs could

be lowered by negotiating contracts for more hospitals. Along with the greater gains in efficiency from participating in larger systems, hospitals and their medical staffs had to give up more of their autonomy with regard to the hospital's operating budget and investment decisions. Only those hospitals faced with financial problems and purchaser pressures for hospital efficiency joined such tightly knit organizations.

The Move toward Vertical Integration

The Effect of Changes in Payment for Medicare Patients

The movement to vertical integration started in the 1980s because of further changes in payment incentives. In 1983 the federal government phased in a fixed price per hospital admission for Medicare patients (DRGs). As hospitals sought to reduce their costs by discharging Medicare patients earlier, they had to find a suitable setting for the aged patient who required additional care. Frequently, the hospital could not find a nursing home to accept that patient. The nursing home might not have a bed available or may have believed that the Medicare payment it would receive would be less than the costs of caring for the particular patient. While the hospital's discharge planner negotiated with each nursing home, the patient remained in the hospital (costing the hospital more money).

It became less costly for many hospitals to buy a nursing home. The hospital would be assured of having a bed available and of the quality of the services provided, and it would not have to engage in protracted negotiations for each patient. These "transactions costs" of negotiating with outside providers and coordinating the care needs of the patient were minimized when the hospital either owned or contracted with a nursing home for a large number of its patients (Conrad and Dowling 1990). The financial incentives of a fixed price per admission caused hospitals to move "downstream" in the acute care production process by contracting with and buying nursing homes.

Medicare payment policy encouraged this vertical integration by separately reimbursing skilled nursing homes and in-home services. By owning a nursing home and a home health agency (or contracting with one), hospitals were able to reduce their inpatient costs as well as receive additional Medicare revenues for care of the patient in the skilled nursing home.

The Effect of Private Insurers

Under pressure from large employers to lower their employees' health insurance premiums, private insurers attempted to lower hospital services— the largest and fastest-increasing portion of their premium. Hospital admissions were reviewed for their appropriateness and insurance benefits were broadened to include diagnostic and surgical services performed in outpatient settings. Utilization review of inpatient admissions and lower-cost substitutes to hospitals dramatically reduced the use of the hospital. Hospital admissions declined 22 percent, from 154 per 1,000 population in 1980, to 121 ten years later. Total patient days fell more rapidly, 24 percent, from 1,159 per 1,000 population in 1980, to less than 880 patient days.

As admissions declined, hospitals moved in two new directions. First, to prevent the loss of revenue from patients being treated in less costly outpatient settings, hospitals began to develop these services themselves. And second, hospitals realized that they needed a larger patient population base upon which to draw.

The Effect of Advances in Medical Technology

The incentive for hospitals to move into outpatient services was reinforced by technological advances in diagnosing and treating patients in outpatient settings. Gallbladder removal used to require a seven-day hospital stay; now it is done on an outpatient basis. Knee surgery, hernia repair, and chemotherapy no longer require inpatient stays. Outpatient surgical procedures have expanded rapidly and now exceed those performed in the hospital. Hospitals are becoming catastrophic care units, where only the most severe cases, such as transplants and gene therapy, will be treated. Less severely ill patients can be treated either in an outpatient setting or in their own home. As the number of inpatients and surgeries declined, outpatient revenues became an important source of hospital revenues.

Interdependency of Hospitals and Physicians

Changes in hospital payment, insurance coverage, and technology increased the interdependency between hospitals and their physicians. The hospital became at risk for physicians' practice patterns. Unless physicians treated inpatients cost-effectively, the hospital would lose money.

Hospitals also depended upon primary care physicians for inpatient referrals and upon specialists to perform their procedures in the hospital's outpatient facilities. Hospitals attempted to lessen their financial risk by monitoring physicians' hospital practice patterns. The hospital tried to expand its population base by increasing the number of physician referrals through "upstream" vertical integration. Some hospitals established ambulatory care clinics, others helped new primary care physicians to locate in their areas, still others developed joint ventures with their physicians to increase their loyalty, and some purchased physicians' practices.

Reinforcing the movement into outpatient surgery and ambulatory care services was the declining profitability of inpatient services. Hospital costs continued to increase as the number of skilled personnel and their wages increased, as more severely ill patients are cared for in the hospital while those who are less costly are treated as outpatients, and as the hospital performs more high-tech services, such as transplants. Hospitals were, however, unable to recover these higher costs by raising prices as they had done previously. Medicare payments and increasing price competition among hospitals limited hospitals' ability to raise their prices. A hospital relying on inpatient services alone could not survive.

The Effect of Capitated Payments

The final stimulus for vertical integration came with the movement toward capitated payments. In areas such as California, the proportion of the population served by HMOs and managed care organizations increased. These organizations receive an annual fee per subscriber and their financial incentive is to minimize the cost of caring for their subscriber population, while not reducing quality. Hospitals not participating in these organizations found themselves competing for a smaller patient population. Thus more hospitals became part of and even started their own HMOs; by doing so, they became completely vertically integrated organizations.

Under capitation, hospitals are no longer profit centers, they become cost centers. Under fee-for-service, hospitals try and increase their admissions. Once the insurance function is added to a delivery system (which are the two parts of an HMO), the delivery system becomes a cost center rather than a revenue center; the organization's goal then is to lower their subscribers' health care costs, such as by reducing hospital use, rather than increase the profitability of each unit within the system.

Capitation contracts require the contracting organization to have a close relationship with one or more medical groups. The medical group, who may receive a percentage of the capitation payment, becomes responsible for providing physician services, monitoring physician quality, and controlling specialist referrals. There is a greater demand for primary care physicians by the medical group, who are needed for managing the patient's treatment under capitation.

The more the payment system moves from fee-for-service to capitation, the greater are the gains from vertical integration. Minimizing the cost of caring for a patient requires close coordination between each of the providers used in treatment. With on-line access to information, a physician treating a patient would have available the patient's history and any drugs that patient is taking. Duplicative tests would not have to be provided and patient information could be forwarded to referral specialists within the same system. As the patient is referred by their primary care physician to labs, x-rays, different specialists, a hospital or surgery center, and in-home health services, neither the patient nor the physician would have to negotiate fees or investigate the availability or quality of the providers being used. The organization would either own these separate entities or have already contracted with them, based on their fees and their performance, such as appropriateness of care.

Advantages of Vertically Integrated Organizations

Efficiency is increased in a coordinated care system. Duplication of tests and other services are reduced, less costly settings are substituted for more costly settings, the patient's treatment process is "managed" for appropriateness, there are economies of scale such as lower costs of capital, and the cost of medical specialists and expensive inpatient services, such as transplants, are more easily controlled once they are part of the same organization. Quality control can also provide the organization with a competitive advantage over insurance companies that have less control over the providers with whom they contract. Similarly, fraud and abuse, which occur when there is limited oversight and information on providers, will be reduced. Liability risk is also lower when providers are monitored and the patient's care is coordinated.

The ability to transfer patient information between providers using uniform records reduces information costs within the organization. More importantly, an information system that follows the patient in different treatment settings, with different providers, as well as over time, enables the organization to better estimate the health care costs of serving different population groups. Information on patient use rates and costs is crucial for estimating insurance premiums for different employee populations.

Vertical integration also makes it possible to achieve reputational economies, such as when an organization (with a good reputation) transfers its reputation to other services it provides, such as a high-quality hospital starting its own nursing home or even its own HMO. It is less costly to transfer a good reputation to a new service than to buy someone else's reputation.

Patient time costs are also lower in a vertically integrated system. It is less costly (in time) for patients to rely on the reputation of a single integrated organization than to gather information on the fees and quality of different providers when ill. The responsibility for monitoring individual providers' quality and for coordinating care is shifted from the patient to the vertically integrated organization. A vertically integrated organization also offers "one-stop shopping." The patient does not have to travel to different locations for referrals, laboratory tests, or pharmacy prescriptions.

As a greater percent of the population moves into managed care organizations, competition is occurring on the basis of premiums, treatment outcomes, and patient convenience. To be competitive, health care organizations need to cover the entire spectrum of health care services, including ambulatory care clinics, family physicians, medical groups, both community and tertiary care hospitals, as well as outpatient care, nursing homes, and home care. Wellness and prevention programs, such as prenatal care, health risk appraisals, and smoking cessation programs, are also included in the integrated spectrum. Wellness and prevention are the most appropriate and least costly way of reducing the usage of expensive acute care services.

Costs of Vertically Integrated Organizations

Vertically integrated organizations as described above have a competitive price, quality, and reputational advantage over other providers and insurers. However, it is costly to develop into such highly integrated organizations. Foremost is the perspective of the providers of care. Under fee-for-service payment, hospitals and other providers increase their revenues by filling their beds and providing additional services. Capitation-based payment systems require the organization's managers to innovate in ways to reduce the use of costly providers, while maintaining quality. Participating providers, both hospitals and medical groups, must have similar cost reduction and quality objectives.

Medical groups must be well integrated into the organization, both philosophically as well as in decision making, if vertical integration is to succeed. Medical groups must be willing to monitor their members for quality, appropriateness of care provided, and productivity. Capitation and salary payments to physicians may lead to decreased work incentives. Unless physicians have incentives or are monitored, physician productivity could decline once in a large group. Yet the close cooperation of medical staffs is often one of the most difficult aspects of developing integrated systems. Physicians are required to surrender part of their autonomy to accept new hospital and specialist referral patterns and review of their practice patterns.

As price (premium) competition for subscribers increases among insurers and HMOs, provider incentives are changing. Traditional (fee-for-service) incentives that reward providers for performing more services increase costs and decrease profitability for capitated organizations. Incentives that emphasize coordination, appropriateness of care, and efficiency are necessary to reward desired behavior among providers in such organizations.

Further, as an organization increases in size and scope of activities, coordination costs become greater and decision making is slower as decisions are pushed to a higher level. Given the greater coordination costs of managing a large and diverse organization, it becomes essential that a sophisticated cost and clinical information system be in place. Such a system will permit management to monitor the cost and clinical performance of each of its entities, evaluate productivity, develop incentive systems for its providers, provide purchasers with treatment outcomes data on their subscribers, and develop accurate data for pricing premiums, which will also minimize the risk of writing insurance.

Summary

The change to Medicare fixed prices, price competition among hospitals, and capitation-based competition changed hospitals' incentives. Technological advances enabled acute care to be moved out of the hospital into other settings, including the patient's home. The benefits of merging with other hospitals to take advantage of economies of scale and diversifying into related services increased. Physician behavior affected a hospital's financial risk, and there was a greater financial interdependence with their medical staff. Health care organizations began to change. Hospitals sought to increase their referral base, to retain the revenues from lower-cost services that substituted for their own services, and to keep all of their referrals within their own system. The size of the organization and the scope of services provided increased. Transactions and coordination costs were reduced when the organization was able to manage these diverse services rather than having the patient or their fee-for-service physician do the coordination.

Payment systems and technology will continue to move health care organizations into becoming more vertically integrated. The structure that will eventually emerge will be one that will minimize coordination costs, provide appropriate incentives, and enhance rapid decision making.

Reference

Conrad, D. A., and W. L. Dowling. "Vertical Integration in Health Services: Theory and Managerial Implications." *Health Care Management Review* 15 (Fall 1990): 9–22.

14

Cost Shifting

Employers and insurers believe that one reason for the rise in employees' health insurance premiums is "cost shifting." When one purchaser, whether it is Medicare, Medicaid, or the uninsured, does not pay their full charges, many believe that hospitals and physicians raise their prices to those who can afford to pay, namely, those with private insurance. Cost shifting is believed to be unfair. Elimination of cost shifting is an important reason why large employers, whose employees have health insurance, favor mandating that all employers provide their employees with health insurance. "All payer" systems, whereby each payer pays the same charges for hospital and medical services, are also favored by those who believe that cost shifting increases their medical prices.

Evidence of cost shifting is based on the observation that different payers pay different prices for similar services. As shown in Table 14.1, Medicaid pays, on average, only 82 percent of costs; Medicare, 88 percent. Other government payers (worker's compensation and civilian dependents of military personnel) pay 100 percent of their costs, while private payers are estimated to pay 130 percent of their costs.

While the logic of cost shifting may seem straightforward, there are a number of troubling questions. For example, can a hospital or physician merely increase its price to those who can pay to recover its losses from those that do not pay? If the provider is able to cost shift, then why do hospitals complain about the uncompensated care they are forced to provide? Further, if the provider is able to offset its losses by increasing its price to those with insurance, why have they not previously done so and thereby earned greater profits?

Table 14.1 Hospitals' Revenues and Costs by Payer, 1991

Payer or Other Source	*Revenues*		*Costs*		
	In Billions of Dollars	*As a Percentage of Total*	*In Billions of Dollars*	*As a Percentage of Total*	*Ratio of Revenues to Costs*
Medicare	76.3	32.8	86.3	38.4	0.88
Medicaid	22.7	9.8	27.8	12.4	0.82
Other government payers	3.2	1.4	3.2	1.4	1.00
Private payers	113.9	49.0	87.8	39.1	1.30
Other	16.4	7.0	19.4	8.7	n.a.

Notes: The data are based on all community hospitals; n.a. = not applicable.
Source: Congressional Budget Office based on analysis by the Prospective Payment Assessment Commission of data from the American Hospital Association's Annual Survey of Hospitals for 1991.

To better understand cost shifting, it is necessary to discuss first the provider's objective when they price their services, and, second, how different objectives result in different pricing strategies.

Setting Prices to Maximize Profits

Firms typically price their services so as to maximize profits, that is, to make as much money as possible. This objective is the simplest one to start with for analyzing hospital and physician price setting. Let us assume that the hospital has two sets of patients, those who can and those who cannot pay for their services. Table 14.2 is used to illustrate how a profit-maximizing price is set for the insured group of patients. The relationship between price (P) and quantity (Q) is inverse, meaning the lower the price the more units are likely to be purchased. Total revenue (TR) is price times quantity. As the price is reduced, more units will be sold and total revenue will increase; after some point, however, the increased number of units sold will not offset the lower price per unit and total revenue will actually decline. The effect on total revenue when price is decreased and more units are sold is shown by the TR curve in Figure 14.1.

To determine the price and output that results in the largest profit, it is also necessary to know what are the costs for producing that output.

Table 14.2   Determining the Profit-Maximizing Price

Price (P)	Quantity (Q)	Total Revenue (TR)	Total Cost (TC)	Profit	TC_2	$Profit_2$
11	1	11	9	2	11	0
10	2	20	13	7	17	3
9	3	27	17	10	23	4
8	4	32	21	11	29	3
7	5	35	25	10	35	0
6	6	36	29	7	41	−5
5	7	35	33	2	47	−12
4	8	32	37	−5	53	−21
3	9	27	41	−14	59	−32

Figure 14.1   The Profit-Maximizing Price with and without a Change in Variable Cost

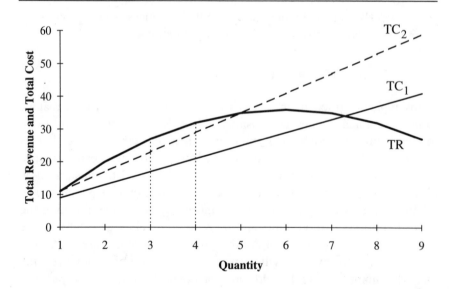

Total cost (TC) consists of two parts, fixed costs, which do not vary as output changes, such as rent for an office or depreciation on a building, and variable costs, which do. For this example, it is assumed that fixed costs are $5 and variable costs are constant at $4 per unit. The difference

between TR and TC is profit. According to Table 14.2, the largest amount of profit occurs when the price is $8 and output equals 4 units. At that price, TR is $32, TC is $21 ($5 fixed cost plus $16 variable costs), and profit is $11.

According to Figure 14.1, the greatest difference between the total cost line (TC) and total revenue, which is profit, is at 4 units of output.

Raising or lowering the price will only reduce profits. If the hospital were to lower its price from $8 to $7, it would have to lower the price on all its units sold. The hospital's volume would increase, total revenue would rise from $32 to $35, or by only $3. Since the variable cost of the extra unit sold is $4, the hospital would lose money on that last unit. The profit at a price of $7 would be $10. Similarly, if the hospital raised its price, from $8 to $9, it would sell one less unit, thereby reducing its variable cost by $4 but it would forgo $5 worth of revenue. Raising its price, once it is at the profit-maximizing price, lowers the hospital's profit.

Table 14.2 illustrates several important points. First, establishing a profit-maximizing price means that the price is set so that the additional revenue received is equal to the additional cost of serving an additional patient. When the change in TR is equal to the change in TC, choosing any other price will result in less profit.

Second, if the hospital's fixed costs were to increase, from $5 to $11, the hospital should not change its price, because if it did, it would make even less profit. With an increase in fixed costs, profit would decline by $6 at every quantity sold. At a price of $8 the firm would still make a total profit of $5—TR is $32 while TC is now $27 ($11 plus $16). If the firm raised its price to $9, to compensate for the rise in its fixed costs, TR would be $27, TC would be $23 ($11 plus $12), and total profit would fall to $4. Thus changes in fixed costs should not affect the firm's profit-maximizing price.

Third, if the hospital's variable costs changed, perhaps because nurses' wages or the cost of supplies increased, then the hospital would find it profitable to change its price. For example, if variable costs increased by $2, and the price-quantity relationship was unchanged, then the largest profit would occur at a price of $9 (TR $-$ TC_2 = Profit$_2$ in Table 14.2). If the price per unit remained at $8 when variable costs increased to $6 per unit, the addition to TR from producing 4 rather than 3 units is only $5. The hospital would lose money on that last unit, whose cost is $6. Thus by raising its price and producing fewer units, the increase in TR slightly exceeds the additional cost of producing that last unit. Hospitals would therefore be expected to raise their prices as their variable costs increased. Similarly, if variable costs were to decline, it would be more profitable for the hospital to lower its price.

The higher variable cost is shown in Figure 14.1 as TC_2. The distance between TR and TC_2, which is profit, is greatest at 3 units of output.

Lastly, hospitals would also be expected to change their prices if the relationship between price and quantity were to change. The price-quantity relationship is a measure of how price-sensitive purchasers are to changes in the hospital's price. When the price is changed and quantity changes by a smaller percentage, purchasers are not very price sensitive; the demand for the hospital's service is *price inelastic.* Conversely, when quantity changes by a greater percentage than the change in price, purchasers are said to be more price sensitive; the demand is *price-elastic.* As the demand for the hospital's services becomes more price sensitive (price elastic), a hospital would be expected to lower its price, even if there were no change in its costs.[1]

For example, if all of a firm's employees have hospital insurance that pays 100 percent of the hospital's charges and permits them to go to any hospital, their demand for hospital services is not very price sensitive. Assume, however, that the hospitals in the area have excess capacity and the employer only permits their employees to go to those hospitals with whom they negotiate the lowest prices. The demand for hospital services would become very price sensitive; a lowering of a hospital's price may cause large increases in its patient volume. Similarly, raising its price, when other hospitals do not, could cause the hospital to lose a great deal of patient volume. Thus a change in the sensitivity of the hospital's price-quantity relationship would change its profit-maximizing price.

If the hospital is already charging a profit-maximizing price to its paying patients and the variable costs of serving paying patients have not changed, then the hospital would make even less profit by further increasing prices to paying patients. Referring to Table 14.2, if the hospital raised its price from \$8 to \$9 simply because other patients did not pay, then the hospital would forgo profit. Assuming the hospital wants to make as much money as possible from those who can afford to pay, then the hospital would not raise its price to those patients unless there was a change in their variable costs or in their price-quantity relationship. Since neither changes when another group of patients pays less, it would not make sense for the hospital to charge its paying patients more.

Based on the above explanation of how a profit-maximizing price is set, changes in prices can be explained by either changes in the variable costs of caring for patients or because of a change in the price sensitivity relationship facing a hospital (or a physician).

Contrary to what many people believe, it is possible that when the government lowers the price it pays for Medicare or Medicaid patients, physicians will *lower* the price they charge to higher-paying patients. For example, assume a physician serves two types of patients, private patients and Medicaid patients. The price charged to Medicaid patients is determined by the government while the physician sets the price for private patients. Traditionally, the price received by the physician for treating private patients is higher than that received for Medicaid patients. The physician presumably allocates his or her time so that revenues per unit of time are the same regardless of the types of patients served. For the return to be equal when the prices for Medicaid and private patients are different, the physician may spend less time on the Medicaid patient.

If the government further reduces the price it pays for Medicaid patients, the physician is likely to decide that he or she can earn more if some of his or her time were shifted away from Medicaid patients toward caring for private patients. As more physicians reduce the time they spend with Medicaid patients and reallocate their time toward the private market, the supply of physician time in this market increases. With an increase in supply, physicians would be willing to reduce their prices to receive an increased number of private patients. Assuming that there is limited demand creation by physicians, a lower price for Medicaid patients is likely to result in lower physician fees for private patients.

Assuming that the objective of both hospitals and physicians is to make as much money as possible, the above two examples suggest that prices for private patients will either be unchanged or reduced when another payer pays the provider less.

Origins of the Claims of Cost Shifting

Based on the above discussion, why then do private purchasers claim that they are being charged more to make up for the lower prices paid by government? The belief that cost shifting is occurring may simply be an artifact of rising trends over time in both hospital prices and uncompensated care. It may appear that hospitals are raising prices to compensate for lower prices to other patients, but in actuality, hospitals' prices to private payers have increased for two reasons: variable costs have been increasing as expenses for wages and supplies have risen and changes in the hospital's payer mix may have enabled them to increase their markups on certain types of private patients. This association of rising prices and uncompensated care does not necessarily indicate a causal relationship.

There is, however, a logical explanation, unrelated to cost shifting, why some purchasers pay more for the same service than other purchasers. Some purchasers might be more price sensitive than others. Previously, private patients had either indemnity insurance or Blue Cross hospital coverage; because of hospitals' close relationship with Blue Cross (hospitals started and controlled Blue Cross), Blue Cross was charged a lower price than indemnity insurers. The price-quantity relationship for those with indemnity insurance represented the average relationship for everyone in the indemnity plan. However, as employers began offering different types of health plans, such as HMOs, PPOs, managed care, in addition to the traditional indemnity plan, and as employees had to pay different premiums and cost sharing under these different plans, the price-quantity relationships of these plans differed. Those with indemnity insurance could choose whatever hospital and physician they desired. Other plans, however, were more restrictive in deciding which providers their subscribers could use. HMOs and PPOs were likely to bargain with providers for lower prices in return for directing their subscribers to these approved providers.

Faced with different price-quantity relationships by these different purchasers, hospitals began charging different prices to each type of payer. These prices take into consideration the price sensitivity of each of these different insurance plans. Those patients remaining in the traditional indemnity plan are being charged the highest prices because they are not restricted in their use of providers. Their insurers cannot promise to direct their subscribers to particular hospitals; they are least able to negotiate lower hospital prices.

Price Discrimination

Charging according to what the market will bear is not really cost shifting; it is simply charging a profit-maximizing price to each group. It is referred to as *price discrimination*. Services have higher markups on those items for which purchasers are willing to pay more. Airlines charge higher prices for first-class seating and lower prices for 21-day advance purchase. Movie theaters charge lower prices for matinees and for senior citizens. Each of these industries is pricing according to these different groups' willingness to pay; each group has a different price-quantity relationship. Hospital pricing is no different. When hospitals place a proportionately higher markup over costs on lab tests or drugs used by inpatients than on the room-and-board fee, this is price discrimination. Patients who have to pay part of the bill themselves can more easily compare hospital room-and-board rates before they enter the hospital. Hospitals therefore have to be price competitive on their room rates. Once a patient is hospitalized, however, patients have little choice in what they pay for services rendered in the hospital. The price-quantity relationships for inpatient services are quite insensitive to prices charged. Hospitals do not face any competition for lab tests or other services provided to their inpatients. Thus their markup for these services is much higher.

Price discrimination is an important reason why some purchasers are able to pay lower hospital prices than others. A large employer or an HMO willing to direct its employees or enrollees to a particular hospital will receive a lower price for the same service than a single patient negotiating with the same hospital. The hospital's price-quantity relationship will be more price sensitive when negotiating with a large purchaser than when the hospital deals with a single insured patient. The single insured patient does not pay higher prices because the large purchaser pays a lower price. The hospital is less concerned with losing one patient's business than it is in losing 1,000 patients from a large purchaser.

Even if the government were to increase its payments to hospitals for treating Medicare patients, the price to the single insured patient would not be reduced because the price-quantity relationship for these patients, which is less price sensitive, would be unchanged. Only if the patient with indemnity insurance became part of a larger purchasing group, who would be willing to offer a hospital a greater volume of patients in return for lower prices, could the indemnity patient receive a lower hospital price. Different prices to different purchasers are related to how price sensitive they are rather than to what other purchasers are paying. As the insurance market has become more segmented, HMOs, PPOs, self-insured employer groups, traditional indemnity-type insurance plans, and so on, hospitals have developed different pricing strategies for each group.

Recent empirical evidence supports the view that hospital prices are not raised to other purchasers when prices are reduced to large purchasers.

Gruber (1992) found that when PPOs received price discounts from hospitals, the hospitals did not increase prices to other paying patients. Instead, the hospital reduced the amount of free or uncompensated care it provided, such as by reducing access to the emergency room, which serves a high proportion of uninsured patients.

Conditions under which Cost Shifting Can Occur

Under certain circumstances, however, it is possible for cost shifting to occur. Some hospitals may have a different pricing objective—they do not price to maximize their profits. These hospitals may voluntarily forgo some profits to maintain good community relationships. When hospitals do not set profit-maximizing prices, then increases in uncompensated care or in their fixed costs may result in the hospital raising its prices to those groups who have a greater ability to pay. For example, "average cost" pricing occurs when a hospital sets its price by relating it to the average cost of caring for all its patients. If one payer (e.g., the government) decides to pay the hospital less, then the average price becomes higher for all other payers. For cost shifting to occur, the purchasers of hospital (or physician) services would also have to be relatively insensitive to the higher prices. If the purchasers were to either switch to other providers or use fewer services as a result of the provider cost shifting to them, the provider's revenues and profits would decline, making cost shifting unprofitable.

One study determined that in 1981 and 1982 Illinois hospitals raised their prices to private patients when the state reduced its Medicaid payments to hospitals (Dranove 1988). In this example, cost shifting did occur.

How likely is it, however, that cost shifting is an important reason why private patients are paying higher medical prices today? Purchasers have become more price sensitive since the mid-1980s. And with the current excess capacity among hospitals and physicians, how likely is it that providers are willing to forgo profits by not setting profit-maximizing prices? Forgoing profits means that the hospital has no better use for those funds. Some ways the hospital could use those higher profits are by purchasing new equipment and starting new services to increase its revenues. New equipment and facilities are also desired by the medical staff, who are an important constituency within the hospital. Paying higher wages also makes it easier to attract needed nursing and technical personnel. Hospitals could enhance their community image and market themselves by providing screening and health awareness programs to their community. And there are the medically indigent. Additional funds could always be used for providing care to those in the community who are unable to afford it and who are not covered by public programs.

It is unlikely that the benefits to the hospital of forgoing profit on some payer group exceeds the benefits to the hospital of using that forgone profit in these other ways. By not setting profit-maximizing prices, the hospital's decision makers are placing a greater weight on benefiting some purchaser group rather than on using those funds for other constituencies.

Cost shifting also occurs when the government pays hospitals a fixed price for Medicare patients' use of the hospital but reimburses outpatient services on a cost basis. If the hospital has $100 in indirect administrative costs to allocate between inpatient units (paid according to a fixed-price DRG) and outpatient units (paid on a cost basis), the hospital will select a cost-allocation method that optimizes its payment from the government, namely, the method that allocates a greater portion of the $100 to outpatient units.

Another type of cost shifting occurs when the government shifts its costs to employers, as when requirements are imposed on employers that would otherwise cost the government money. For example, if the government required all employers to buy health insurance for their employees, such an employer mandate would reduce the government's Medicaid expenditures for low-income employees and their dependents.

Summary

Previously, when insurance premiums were paid almost entirely by the employer and managed care was not yet popular, hospitals were probably less interested in making as much money as possible. Many were reimbursed according to their costs and they could achieve many of their goals without having to set profit-maximizing prices. However, as occupancy rates declined, leaving hospitals with excess capacity, price competition increased, HMOs and PPOs entered the market, and hospitals could no longer count on having their costs reimbursed, regardless of what those costs were. Hospital profitability declined. Those hospitals that did not price so as to make as much money as possible began to do so. Some cost shifting occurred.

The cost of providing hospital services has continued to increase, new technology has made possible more costly treatments, such as transplants, and hospitals have had to raise their prices to cover these increased costs. At the same time, the discount from charges has become larger as Medicare and Medicaid pay hospitals a smaller percent of the hospital's charges. And price competition among hospitals has limited the ability of the hospital to receive its full list prices. As more of the insured population moves into more restrictive health plans, those remaining in indemnity-type plans are less price sensitive. Thus as hospitals establish prices according to each payer group's price sensitivity, those in the more traditional indemnity plans, who are less price sensitive, pay more for the same services than those in health plans with greater purchasing power.

Differences in hospital prices for different payer groups today is more likely the result of price discrimination than cost shifting. The difference between these two explanations is significant. Even if others, such as the government, were to pay more, prices for private patients would not decline.

Note

1. The effect of price sensitivity on hospital prices and markups is based on the following formula:

markup = (1/price sensitivity) × 100 percent

Thus if a hospital believes that the price sensitivity of a particular employee group is such that a 1 percent increase in the hospital's price leads to a 1 percent decline in admissions, then the hospital's markup would be 100 percent [(1/1) × 100]. If use of services were more price sensitive, such that a 1 percent price increase leads to a 3 percent decline in admissions, then the markup would be 33 percent [(1/3) × 100]. If the hospital's costs of serving the patients were the same in both examples, then depending upon their price sensitivity, the prices charged to each employee group could vary greatly.

References

Gruber, J. "The Effect of Price Shopping in Medical Markets: Hospital Responses to PPOs in California." Working Paper No. 4190. Cambridge, MA: National Bureau of Economic Research, Inc., 1992.

Dranove, D. "Pricing by Non-Profit Institutions: The Case of Hospital Cost-Shifting." *Journal of Health Economics* 7 (March 1988): 48–49.

15

Can Price Controls Limit
Medical Expenditure Increases?

In the debate over health care reform, proponents of regulation, such as those who favor a single-payer system, have proposed placing controls on the prices physicians and hospitals charge so as to limit the rise in medical expenditures. Then, to prevent hospitals and physicians from circumventing such controls simply by performing more services, they would also impose an overall limit (a "global budget") on total medical expenditures.

Price controls and global budgets may seem to be obvious approaches for limiting rising medical expenditures, but the potential consequences should be examined before placing one-seventh of the U.S. economy (which is approaching a trillion dollars a year) under government control. The health care industry in the United States is larger than the economies of most countries in the world. An announcement in any country that price conrols would be imposed on the entire economy would seem incredible to all who have observed the economies of Eastern Europe and Russia this decade. Widespread shortages occurred, many of the goods produced were of shoddy quality, and black markets developed. In these countries, the inherent failures of a controlled economy have been recognized, and now their task is to try to develop free markets.

Why should we think health care is so different that access to care, high quality, and innovation can be achieved better by price controls and regulation than by reliance on competitive markets? What consequences

151

are likely if price controls are imposed on medical services? (For a more complete discussion on this subject, see Haislmaier 1993.)

Effect of Price Controls in Theory

Imbalances between Supply and Demand

Imbalances between demands for care and supply of services will occur. The demand for medical services and the cost of providing those services are constantly changing. Prices bring about an equilibrium between the demanders and suppliers in a market. Prices reflect changes in demands or in the costs of producing a service. When demands increase (perhaps because of an aging population or rising incomes), prices will increase. Higher prices will cause some of the demand to decrease, but suppliers will respond to the higher prices by increasing the quantity of their services. Higher prices provide a signal (and an incentive) to suppliers that greater investment in personnel and equipment will be needed to meet the increased demand.

When regulators initially place controls on prices, they are assuming that the conditions that brought about the initial price, namely the demands for service and the costs of producing that service, will not change. However, these do change, for many reasons. Thus the controlled price will no longer be an equilibrium price. The problem with price controls is that demand is constantly changing, as is the cost of providing services. While regulators often allow some increases in prices each year to adjust for inflation, seldom, if ever, are these price increases sufficient to reflect the changes in demand or costs that are occurring. When prices are not flexible, an imbalance between demand and supply will occur.

Not only do the demands and costs of producing services change, but the "product" itself, that is, medical care, is continually changing, complicating the picture for regulators. For example, the population is aging. Thus, if the hospital treats more seriously ill patients, the hospital is forced to spend more resources on those patients, such as providing more nursing time and more tests. Relatively new diseases, such as AIDS, require extensive testing, treatment, and prolonged care. Technology is continuing to improve. In the last ten years, transplants have become commonplace, and they are occurring more frequently. Diagnostic equipment has reduced the need for many exploratory surgeries. Low-birthweight infants can now survive. Such continuing advances increase the demands for medical services and require a greater use of skilled labor, expensive monitoring equipment, and new imaging machines. Unless regulators are aware of these changes in the medical "product" and technology, their controlled prices will be below the costs of providing these services. How will these demands then be met? Imbalances will undoubtedly occur because regulators cannot anticipate all of the changes in demands, costs, and technology.

Shortages

Shortages are the inevitable consequence of price controls. Demands for medical services are continually increasing, yet price controls limit increases in supply. To expand its services, a hospital or a medical group must be able to attract additional employees by increasing wages to lure skilled and trained employees away from their current employers. Similarly, as wages increase, trained nurses who are not currently employed as nurses will find it financially attractive to return to nursing, and more people will choose nursing careers as wages become comparable to those in other professions. However, if hospitals cannot raise wages because they cannot raise their prices, they will not be able to hire the necessary nurses needed to expand their services.

Price controls not only limit increases in medical services but they actually cause a reduction in such services, which exacerbates the shortage over time. As prices and wages continue to increase throughout the economy, price controls on the health sector make it difficult for hospitals and medical groups to pay competitive wages and to pay rising supply costs. Hospitals must hire nurses and technicians, buy supplies, pay heating and electric bills, and replace or repair equipment. A hospital that cannot pay competitive wages will be unable to retain its employees. If the wages of hospital accountants are not similar to those of accountants working in nonhospital settings, fewer accountants will choose to work in hospitals—or those who do accept lower wages may not be, in general, as well qualified. As medical costs increase faster than the permitted increases in prices, hospitals and medical groups will be unable to retain their existing labor force and provide its current services.

As costs per patient rise faster than government controlled prices, hospitals, outpatient facilities, and physicians' practices are faced with two choices: they can either care for fewer, more costly patients, or they can care for the same number of patients but devote fewer resources to each patient.

Eliminating all the waste in the current system would result merely in a one-time savings. If rising expenditures were caused by new technologies, aging of the population, and new diseases, and not by waste, medical costs still would rise faster than the rate at which hospitals and other providers were being reimbursed. Providers then would be faced with the same two choices: that is, either caring for fewer patients or devoting fewer resources to each patient and thus providing a lower quality of service.

Price controls on medical services cause the demand for medical services to exceed the supply. The out-of-pocket price the patient pays for a physician visit, an MRI, an ultrasound, and lab tests will rise more slowly than if the price were not controlled. (The "real", or inflation-adjusted, price to the patient is likely to fall.) Consequently, even though the demand by patients for such services increases, suppliers cannot increase their services if the cost of doing so exceeds the fixed price. In fact, over time, the shortage will become even larger, since the fixed price will cover the cost of fewer such services. We have seen this occur when rent controls were imposed on housing, such as in New York. The demand for rent-controlled housing continually exceeds its supply, and the supply of existing housing decreases as the costs of upkeep exceed the allowable increases in rent. Indeed, landlords have abandoned entire city areas.

Shift of Capital away from Price-Controlled Services

Further, since profitability is reduced on services subject to price control, capital investment will eventually be shifted to areas that are not subject to control and in which they can earn higher returns. Less private capital will be available for the development of HMOs, investment in computer technology for patient care management, and research and development toward breakthrough drugs. Price controls on hospitals cause hospital investment to decline and capital to move into nonregulated outpatient services and home health services. Should all health services become subject to controls, then capital would move to nonhealth industries and to geographic regions without controls.

Effects of Price Controls in Practice

Medicaid

Price controls have been tried rather extensively, both in this country as well as in others. Shortages and decreased access to care, which typify the Medicaid program, are caused by price controls. Once a patient is eligible for Medicaid, the price he or she has to pay for medical services is greatly reduced, thus increasing their demand for such services. Medicaid payments to physicians are fixed, however, and below what physicians could earn by serving non-Medicaid patients. Low provider payments have decreased the profitability of serving Medicaid patients and resulted in a shortage of Medicaid services. As the difference increases between prices for Medicaid and private patients, more of the physician's time is shifted toward serving private patients, thereby increasing the shortage of medical services faced by Medicaid patients.

Medicare

Hospitals are also subject to price controls on the payments they receive from Medicare. When fixed prices per diagnostic admission were introduced in 1984, hospitals began to code their Medicare patients' diagnoses to maximize their reimbursements. Medicare hospital payments increased sharply, and 75 percent of the increase was attributed to "code creep." Eventually, the government tightened up on Medicare payments so much that now more than two-thirds of all hospitals lose money on their Medicare patients. Consequently, anecdotal evidence suggests that hospitals "dump" on other hospitals their Medicare patients whose costs exceed their payments.

When price controls and actual fee reductions recently were imposed on Medicare physician fees, physicians whose fees were reduced most have shown the largest increases in the volume of their services. For example, radiologists' fees declined by 12 percent, while their volume increased by 13 percent. Similarly, urologists' fees declined 5 percent, while their volume increased 12 percent. These specialists were apparently able to "create demand" among their Medicare fee-for-service patients.

Rationing

Under price controls, as demands for medical services exceed supplies, what criteria will be used to ration the available supplies? Undoubtedly, emergency cases would take precedence over elective services, but how would elective services be rationed? In some countries where age is a criterion, those above a certain age do not have access to hip replacements, kidney dialysis, heart surgery, and other services. Both the quality of life and life expectancy would be reduced.

Waiting Lists

Typically, waiting lists are used for rationing elective procedures. In other countries that rely on this approach, waiting times for surgical procedures, whether for cataracts or open-heart surgery, may vary from 6 months to 2 years. Delays are costly in terms of reduced quality of life and in life expectancy. When resources are limited, acute care has a higher priority than preventive services. Women over the age of 50 have a lower use rate of mammograms in Canada, where price controls and global budgets are used, than in the state of Washington (Katz et al. 1992).

Those who can afford to wait, that is, those with lower time costs, such as the retired, will be more likely to receive physician services than those with higher time costs. Access to nonemergency physician services will be determined by the value patients place on their time. Waiting is costly in that it uses productive resources (or enjoyable time). There is a large, but less visible, cost associated with waiting. Suppose the out-of-pocket price of a physician's office visit is limited to $10, but the patient must take 3 hours off work to wait and see the physician. If the patient earns $20 an hour, the effective cost of that visit is $70. The "lower" costs of a price-controlled system never include the lost productivity to society or the value of that time to the patient. Patients with high time costs would be willing to pay not to wait, but they do not have that option. They cannot buy medical services whose value exceeds what they would be willing to pay.

The effects of price controls are often a greater burden on those with low incomes and on those who do not know how to work the system. Those with connections frequently are seen more quickly by specialists, and those with higher incomes can travel elsewhere to receive care. For example, in 1990, the premier of Quebec received cancer treatment in the United States at his own expense (Wood 1990).

Deterioration of Quality

As the costs of providing medical services increase faster than the controlled price, providers may reduce the resources used in treatment, resulting in a deterioration of quality. A physician may prefer a highly sophisticated diagnostic test such as magnetic resonance imaging, but to conserve resources he or she may order an x-ray instead. The value to the patient of a diagnostic test may exceed its cost, but an overall limit on costs will preclude performing many cost-beneficial tests or procedures.

Experience with Medicaid confirms these concerns with quality of care. Large numbers of patients are seen for very short visits in Medicaid "mills." Such short visits are more likely to lead to incorrect diagnoses and treatment. Similarly, in Japan, where physicians' fees are controlled, Japanese physicians see an average of 49 patients a day, and 13 percent see 100 patients a day (Ikegami 1991).

When controlled prices do not reflect differences among hospitals or physicians, suppliers have less incentive to provide higher-quality services. If all physicians are paid the same fee, there may be no incentive to invest the time to become board certified. In a price-controlled environment with excess demand, even low-quality providers can survive and prosper. Similarly, drug and equipment manufacturers have no incentive to invest in higher-quality products if such products could not be priced to reflect their higher value.

Gaming the System

Price controls provide incentives for providers to try and "game" the system to increase their revenues. For example, physicians paid fee-for-service are likely to decrease the time they devote to each visit, which enables the physician to see more patients, and thus bill for more visits. Less physician time per patient represents a more hurried visit and, presumably, lower-quality care. Also, physicians are likely to "unbundle" their services; by dividing a treatment or visit into its separate parts, they could charge for each part separately. For example, separate visits may be scheduled for diagnostic tests, to receive the results of those tests, and to receive medications. Price controls also provide physicians and hospitals with an incentive to "upcode" the type of services they provide, that is, to bill a brief office visit as a comprehensive exam.

Gaming the system results in increased regulatory costs, because a larger bureaucracy is needed to administer and monitor compliance with price controls. C. Jackson Grayson, who was in charge of price controls that were imposed in the United States in 1971, stated, "We started Phase II [from 1971 to 1973] with 3½ pages of regulations and ended with 1,534" (*Wall Street Journal* March 29, 1993, p. 14).

Gaming is also costly to patients. Multiple visits to the physician, to enable the physician to bill for each visit separately, increases patient travel and waiting times. It is an inefficient use of the patient's time and may discourage patients from using needed services.

Global Budgets

To ensure that gaming does not increase total expenditures, an expenditure limit (global budget) is often superimposed on price controls. Included in a global budget are all medical expenditures for hospital and physician services, outpatient and inpatient care, health insurance and HMO premiums, and consumer out-of-pocket payments. Unless the global budget is comprehensive, expenditures and investments will shift to nonregulated sectors. Additional controls will then be imposed to prevent expenditure growth in these areas, and monitoring compliance with the controls becomes even more costly.

What happens under global budgets when demand for certain providers or managed care organizations increases? The more-efficient HMOs cannot increase their number of physicians and facilities to meet increased enrollment demands. Thus, the public is precluded from choosing the more-efficient, more-responsive health plans that are subject to overall budget limits. Limiting a physician's total physician revenue discourages the use of physician assistants and nurse practitioners, although they could increase the physician's productivity because the physician would prefer receiving the revenue rather than sharing it. Once a physician has reached the overall revenue limit, what incentive does he or she have to continue serving patients? Why not work fewer hours and take longer vacations? What incentives do hospitals or physicians have to develop innovative, less costly delivery systems, such as managed care, outpatient diagnostics and surgery, or home infusion programs, if the funds must be taken from existing programs and providers?

Efficient providers are penalized if they cannot spend increased expenditures to expand, and patients lose the opportunity to be served by more efficient providers.

Will a hospital that is about to exceed its overall budget be forced to close its doors? Hospitals adjust to stringent budget limits by keeping patients longer, since long-stay patients require fewer resources than performing procedures on more patients. Tight limits will result in greater delays in admitting patients, and patients will have less access to beneficial but costly technology.

Global budgets are based on the assumption that the government knows the exact "right" amount of medical expenditures for the nation. However, there is no correct percent of GNP that should go for medical care and the fact that other countries spend less than the United States does not tell us which country we should emulate, nor what we should forgo. Medical expenditures increase for many reasons. No accurate information exists as to how much of the rise in expenditures is due to waste, new diseases (such as AIDS), an aging population, and new technology. The quality of health care will deteriorate, and there will be long waiting lines for treatment if price controls and global budgets were set too low.

It is questionable whether in the face of shortages and complaints about access to medical services politicians would permit a strict global budget to continue. More likely, politicians would respond to their constituents' complaints and relax the budget limit. This has, in fact, occurred in other countries when access to medical services became too limited because of price controls and global budgets. Great Britain, for example, permits "buyouts." A private medical market is allowed to develop, and those with higher incomes who can afford to buy private medical insurance jump the queue to receive medical services from private providers. To the extent that buyouts are permitted, medical expenditures will increase more rapidly and a two-tier system will evolve. If a buyout is envisaged, then the rationale for price controls and global budgets is questionable.

Summary

Price controls and global budgets provide the appearance of controlling rising prices and expenditures, but in reality, they lead to cheating and a reduction in quality, impose large costs upon patients and providers, and do little to improve efficiency.

If the purpose of regulation is to improve efficiency, eliminate inappropriate services, and decrease the costly duplication of medical technology, then government policies should provide incentives to achieve these goals. Such incentives are more likely to occur in a system where purchasers make cost-conscious choices and providers must compete for those purchasers. Competitive systems provide both purchasers and providers with incentives to weigh the benefits and costs of new medical technology. When patients are willing to pay not to wait and to have access to new technology, medical expenditures will increase faster, but the rate of increase would be more appropriate.

References

Haislmaier, E. F. "Why Global Budgets and Price Controls Will Not Curb Health Costs." Washington, DC: The Heritage Foundation, 1993.

Ikegami, N. "Japanese Health Care—Low Cost through Regulated Fees." *Health Affairs* 10 (Fall 1991): 87–109.

Katz, S., E. B. Larson, and J. P. LoGerfo. "Trends in the Utilization of Mammography in Washington State and British Columbia." *Medical Care* 30 (April 1992): 320–28.

Wood, N. "Missing, But Not Forgotten." *McLean's* 103 (10 December 1990): 14.

16

Managed Care Competition

An important policy debate concerns the organization and delivery of medical services—namely, should this country rely on regulation of hospital and physician expenditures or on competition among managed care organizations to achieve efficiency in the provision of medical services? Or has the competitive approach been tried and failed, as its critics claim? To discuss these issues, it is necessary, first, to discuss what is meant by managed care competition, and, second, what is the evidence to date on how well managed care competition has performed.

What Is Managed Care?

Managed care is an attempt to intervene in the delivery of medical services to eliminate unnecessary and inappropriate services, without reducing quality, thereby reducing the cost of providing medical treatment. The approaches used by managed care organizations (MCOs) to intervene in the delivery of medical services vary in the degree to which they both intervene in medical decision making and also restrict the patient's choice of provider.

The least restrictive, less interventionist, form of managed care is utilization review, such as prior authorization for hospital admission. At the other end of the spectrum, a patient's choice of physician may be limited by having to choose a primary care physician from among a panel of physicians, a "gatekeeper," who must first be consulted before the patient can receive approval for a referral to a specialist. Typically, utilization review requires approval for a hospital admission, and once admitted, the patient's length of stay is reviewed to make sure his or her stay does not exceed what is medically necessary. Retrospective review of the treatment is undertaken to ensure that it was appropriate. Catastrophic case managers, now included in most managed care organizations, intervene once a patient's medical expenses exceed a certain threshold, with the objective of reducing the costs of the medical treatment in a manner that is satisfactory to the patient and their family.

Managed care organizations also differ in the extent to which they limit or encourage patients to use a select network of providers. Some MCOs use closed provider panels, and patients using nonpanel providers must either pay the full cost or a percentage of the cost themselves. The most familiar type of MCO is the health maintenance organization (HMO); it relies upon a select group of providers, and the patient is responsible for the full costs of going outside the provider network. A point-of-service (POS) plan is an HMO that permits its enrollees to use non-HMO providers by paying a high copayment each time they use such providers. Preferred provider organizations (PPOs) typically use utilization review and provide patients with financial incentives to use PPO providers, such as lower copayments. Managed fee-for-service indemnity insurance plans have the fewest restrictions on the patient's choice of provider and rely on utilization review techniques to limit medical expenditures.

Figure 16.1 shows the movement away from unmanaged fee-for-service toward managed care. As of 1990, only 5 percent of employees were in unmanaged care, a decline from 41 percent in 1987, only a few years ago. The most popular form of managed care is managed fee-for-service, which permits greater choice of provider than permitted by HMOs and PPOs.

Managed care techniques that relied on utilization review to reduce hospital admissions were able to achieve large savings (Feldstein, Wickizer, and Wheeler 1988). To receive additional savings, managed care has moved into new areas, such as substituting in-home services for continued care in the hospital, instituting prescription drug formularies, reducing inappropriate surgical procedures (as much as 30 percent of some are considered to be inappropriate), and reducing variations in physicians' practice styles.

Managed care organizations also vary in the degree to which they rely on financial incentives to encourage their participating physicians

Figure 16.1 The Trend toward Managed Care

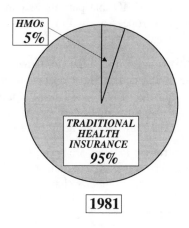

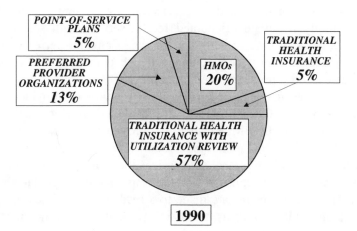

Health Maintenance Organization (HMO): An organization that provides comprehensive health care services to a voluntarily enrolled membership for a prepaid fee. An HMO controls costs through stringent utilization management, payment incentives to its physicians, and restricted access to its providers.

Preferred Provider Organization (PPO): A third party payer contracts with a group of medical providers that agrees to furnish services at negotiated fees in return for prompt payment and a guaranteed patient volume. PPOs control costs by keeping fees down and curbing excessive service through utilization management.

Figure 16.1   Continued

Point-of-Service (POS): An HMO that permits its enrollees access to nonparticipating providers if the enrollees are willing to pay a high copayment each time they use such providers.

Traditional Health Insurance with Utilization Review (UR): Fee-for-service payment to providers, annual deductible and copayment by patients, plus utilization review, which consists of review of hospital utilization to evaluate the appropriateness, necessity, and quality of care provided. Preadmission certification, concurrent review, and retrospective review are part of the UR process.

Traditional Health Insurance: Patients are permitted to go to any provider and the provider is paid fee-for-service. The patient normally pays a small annual deductible plus 20 percent of the provider's charge, up to an annual out-of-pocket limit of $3,000.

---

and hospitals to provide medical services in an efficient manner. Some MCOs simply negotiate discounted fee-for-service with selected providers. Others pay their providers a capitation amount per enrollee and thereby place their providers at financial risk if their patient's medical expenses exceed a predetermined amount.

The degree to which the MCO must monitor its providers varies according to how those providers are paid and whether they are at financial risk. In some HMOs, where the providers are paid a salary and are not at risk, the HMO monitors its medical providers to ensure that the physicians are productive, that the services they provide are appropriate, and that they are not high users of lab tests or other medical services. When capitation payments are made to a medical group, then the group is at risk and will monitor its members' medical decision making.

The managed care plan provides its enrollees with a set of medical benefits in return for an annual premium (usually paid in monthly installments). If the required medical services for an enrollee group exceeds their premiums, the health plan is at risk for the difference. Similarly, the health plan receives the profit if the premiums exceed the required services. The premium in a typical MCO is allocated as shown in Figure 16.2. The ABC Managed Care Health Plan retains 15 percent of the premium to cover expenses associated with marketing, administration, and profit. Forty percent of the premium is allocated for hospital and other medical facility expenses; another 40 percent is set aside for physician services; and 5 percent is allocated for pharmacy

Figure 16.2 Allocation of the Premium Dollar by HMOs

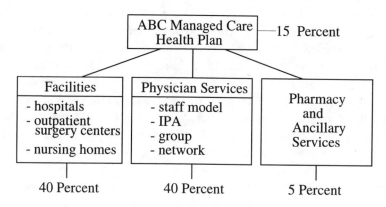

Types of HMOs:

Staff Model: An HMO that delivers health services through a physician group that is controlled by the HMO unit.

IPA: An HMO that contracts directly with physicians in independent practices.

Group: An HMO that contracts with one independent group practice to provide health services.

Network: An HMO that contracts with two or more independent group practices.

and ancillary services. Use of services by enrollees outside of the plan area and certain catastrophic expenses may also be included in the health plan's percentage.

Providers within each of these budgetary allocations may be paid in one of several ways. For example, some managed care organizations place their physicians on a salary, others pay discounted fee-for-service, and still others capitate their physicians (pay an annual amount to the physician group for each enrollee for whom they are responsible). Within each of these payment arrangements a certain percentage of the budget allocation is withheld to ensure that there are sufficient funds available to provide all the necessary services. Funds remaining at the end of the year are then divided among the members of that provider group and the health plan.

More MCOs are beginning to shift the risk from the health plan to the providers. By capitating the medical and hospital groups within the MCO, the health plan is able to shift part of the risk (and profit) to the providers. As this occurs, it is up to each provider group to carefully monitor the performance (both use and quality of services) of its participating providers.

When providers within an MCO are placed at financial risk, they have more incentive to perform "too few" services than if they were paid discounted fee-for-service. Monitoring participating physicians and hospitals according to the quality of care provided and the enrollees' satisfaction is essential for any managed care plan. Poor performance by a few providers could cause financial ruin to the reputation of a health plan. Given the competition by other managed care plans, it becomes crucial for MCOs to compete on the basis of patient satisfaction and quality of care, as well as on their premiums. Employers (particularly larger ones) are becoming sophisticated purchasers of medical services and are requesting data from MCOs on the cost of caring for their employees, quality of care provided, and outcome measures.

How Well Has Managed Care Competition Performed?

In response to critics that market competition has been tried and that it doesn't work, proponents of market competition counter that it has not really been tried. A significant portion of the population is excluded from competitive pressures. Those eligible for Medicare and Medicaid have limited price incentives to enroll in managed care plans. Less than 8 percent of the more than 32 million aged and less than 10 percent of the 15.4 million on Medicaid are signed up in HMOs. An additional 35 million are uninsured. Managed care systems, therefore, do not compete for approximately 80 million, or 32 percent, of the U.S. population who rely on the fee-for-service system (Congressional Budget Office 1992, 26, Table A-1).

The new competitive pressures in medical services are therefore directed at the remaining 68 percent of the population, who primarily have employer-purchased health insurance. However, even within this population, managed care systems have not been forced to compete on price (premiums). Important to the success of the managed care competition strategy is that employees make cost-conscious choices among competing health plans. If an employee does not have to pay any part of a health plan's premium, he or she is likely to choose the health plan that offers the maximum amount of choice, the highest perceived quality, the lowest out-of-pocket expenses, and the richest set of benefits. When the employee is not required to make any trade-off between the value he or she places on additional services and their additional cost, MCOs will compete on services, not on their premiums.

There are several reasons why employees do not make cost-conscious choices when selecting their health plan. First, many employers contribute either the entire premium, regardless of which plan is selected, or their contribution exceeds the premium of the lowest-cost health plan offered to their employees. According to a Bureau of Labor Statistics survey, 54 percent of employers in 1989 paid the entire premium for single employees and 34 percent of employers did so for employees with families. These proportions were higher in earlier years. When the employer pays the entire premium, the employee has no incentive to choose a less-expensive health plan.

Even in those cases where the employer does not pay the entire premium, many employers' contributions exceed the cost of the lowest-cost health plan offered. Thus the employer contribution distorts the employee's choice of health plan. Employers often contribute a flat dollar amount toward the employees' health insurance premium based on the average premiums of all the health plans offered, or the amount contributed may cover the entire premium of the HMO and most of the premium of the indemnity plan.

Second, the savings from choosing a lower-priced health plan are taxed, in that the employee receives the savings in the form of higher wages, while employer funds spent on additional health plan benefits are not. Many high-income employees would rather have their before-tax income spent on more-expensive health plans with smaller deductibles and copayments. It is for this reason that higher-income employees are reluctant to choose health plans that offer stringent cost-containment features and restricted provider groups. The after-tax savings have been insufficient to justify the increased inconvenience.

When employees have to pay the additional premium cost for choosing a more-expensive health plan, they will have to decide whether the value of a health plan that offers unrestricted choice of providers is worth the extra cost.

To date, market competition among MCOs has been quite limited because managed care competition has not been available to many and when it has, employees have not had to make cost-conscious choices.

Even with these disincentives for employees to balance the higher cost of health plans and the additional value of those benefits, a number of studies have shown that managed care techniques and HMOs lower hospital use rates and total medical costs (U.S. Congressional Budget

Office 1992, 6–7). The early forms of MCOs were HMOs, who had lower hospital utilization rates than traditional fee-for-service indemnity plans. As enrollment in HMOs increased and threatened their market share, traditional indemnity plans responded by introducing utilization review.

Between 1980 and 1990, hospital admissions per 1,000 persons declined from 145 to 138, or 5 percent. However, hospital patient days per 1,000 persons declined from 1,206 to 907, or 25 percent (with the result that hospital occupancy decreased from 75.6 to 66.8). In states where there is a great deal of managed care competition, such as California, there were 102 hospital admissions per 1,000 in 1990, which is 26 percent lower than the U.S. average, and patient days per 1,000 in California in 1990 were 624, or 31 percent lower than the U.S. average. As other states approach the degree of managed care competition that exists in California, large reductions in use rates are likely to occur.

A more accurate indication of the effects of competition has been the changes in total per capita medical costs, which is a broader measure than just hospital utilization. Figure 16.3 compares the annual percent increase in per capita health expenditures from 1980 to 1991 in California, which has a high proportion of its population enrolled in managed care plans, to the average for the United States, as well as to several states that rely more on regulation to control rising health care expenditures. According to these data, managed care competition in California has resulted in a much lower annual rate of increase in per capita health costs than occurred in more-regulated states.

"Managed Care Competition" versus "Managed Competition"

There is disagreement among those who want a competitive managed care system. There are those who believe that limiting employer tax-free contributions for health insurance to the lowest-cost health plan will be sufficient to encourage employees to make cost-conscious choices among health plans. Others believe that the health care market must also be "managed" by using an intermediary organization, a health insurance purchasing cooperative (HIPC) for a specified geographic area. *Managed competition* involves "active collective purchasing agents contracting with health care plans on behalf of a large group of subscribers and continuously structuring and adjusting the market to overcome attempts to avoid price competition" (Enthoven 1993). There is thus a difference between managed care competition and managed competition.

Figure 16.3   Average Annual Growth in Per Capita Health
Expenditures by Selected States, 1980–1991

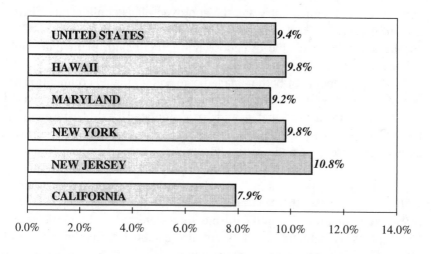

UNITED STATES	9.4%
HAWAII	9.8%
MARYLAND	9.2%
NEW YORK	9.8%
NEW JERSEY	10.8%
CALIFORNIA	7.9%

0.0%   2.0%   4.0%   6.0%   8.0%   10.0%   12.0%   14.0%

Note: Figures are for expenditures on hospital care, physician services, and prescription drug purchases in retail outlets.
Source: Kathy Cowan, Health Care Financing Administration, Office of the Actuary (Washington, DC).

The advocates of managed, or regulated, competition do not trust unregulated competition to achieve the desired outcomes. They propose to limit consumer choice to a standard benefit package, chosen by a national board, which would eliminate competition among health plans who would otherwise design their benefit packages to appeal to better-risk groups. They also favor the formation of HIPCs as purchasers to be able to spread risk, take advantage of economies in administration, and exercise purchasing power over competing health plans.

There is concern, however, that the standard benefit package under managed competition will be subject to politics and include more benefits than many are willing to purchase.

There is the further concern that HIPCs might actually *reduce* competition by limiting the number of health plans that are able to compete for HIPC enrollees. Once the winning health plans are selected by the HIPC, the losing plans will find it difficult to reenter the market. HIPC-approved health plans would thereby be protected from the competition of excluded plans. Excess capacity (of health plans) is eliminated and future negotiations between the HIPC and health plans will be similar to public utility regulation. If the approved health plans "capture" the HIPC (as often occurs with producers and their regulatory agencies), competitors are denied entry and the approved plans could act as a cartel and limit access to technology, to limit their premium increases. HIPC enrollees would be unable to choose non-HIPC health plans that might better serve them.

The proponents of both managed care and regulated competition are very concerned by the Clinton administration's use of the term "managed competition" to install what would be a regulated health care environment. The proposed standard benefit package was very comprehensive, as was predicted, and the proposed purchasing cooperatives (renamed "health alliances") would become monopolies within a state, requiring most of the state's population to join. These alliances would then contract with just a few health plans and, because of their enormous size and proposed regulations, would be able to dictate terms to participating health plans. A national board would also establish a maximum rate of increase in each state's health expenditures.

The Clinton administration proposal is far removed from the conditions necessary for competition to occur and for its desired outcomes to be achieved. If consumers do not agree with the policies and preferences of the health alliance, they cannot join other health plans. Health plans are precluded from competing for subscribers unless they agree to the terms established by the single purchaser. And enrollees and health plans are unable to spend more on medical services and technology if such expenditures exceed the increase in the national board's approved rate increase. The concepts of choice, willingness to pay, and competition have been eliminated from the administration's proposal.

Summary

Unless managed care plans are able to compete for employees according to their premiums, availability of services, quality of care and outcomes measures, and enrollee satisfaction, they will not have an incentive to be efficient and innovative in providing medical services. Employees will be denied the choice of being able to choose between lower premiums and greater access. No other method of organizing the delivery of medical services, such as regulation of hospital and physician fees and expenditures, will produce incentives for achieving the desired outcomes.

Critics of managed care competition claim that managed care will not reduce the rise in medical expenditures as much as arbitrary expenditure limits, as exist in Canada. That is probably correct. If they wanted to, managed care plans could act like the government in limiting their enrollees' access to medical services, specialists, and to new technology. Managed care plans, however, are subject to competition from other managed care plans. If too tight a limit is placed on patient access and satisfaction, a managed care plan would lose enrollees who are willing to pay more to join health plans that are less stringent on access.

When government reduces access through an arbitrary expenditure limit, it does not have to be concerned with patients switching to another health system, particularly when private systems are prohibited, as occurs in Canada and in the administration's health care proposal. Under such regulated systems the government achieves its savings, not by greater efficiency, but by regulating fees and hospital rates below what would occur in a competitive market. The consequence is higher patient "costs," in terms of reduced patient access, as providers reduce their supply of services.

Managed care competition will not solve the problem of the uninsured. Assuring universal access to care is a financing problem. It is the obligation of society and government, not the providers of medical services, to enable those with low incomes to purchase adequate health insurance. Once the government subsidizes medical care for the poor, managed care competition's role is to provide those services efficiently and satisfactorily.

References

Enthoven, A. C. "The History and Principles of Managed Competition." *Health Affairs* 12 (Supplement 1993): 29.

Feldstein, P. J., T. Wickizer, and J. R. C. Wheeler. "Private Cost Containment: The Effects of Utilization Review Programs on Health Care Use and Expenditures." *New England Journal of Medicine* 318 (19 May 1988): 1310–14.

U.S. Congressional Budget Office. *The Potential Impact of Certain Forms of Managed Care on Health Care Expenditures*. Washington, DC: U.S. Congressional Budget Office, 1992.

17

American Competitiveness
and Rising Health Costs

One of the oft-cited reasons for controlling the rise in health care costs is that it makes American business less competitive internationally. Automobile executives, for example, complain that their competitors in other countries have lower health care costs per employee, thereby enabling them to sell their products at a lower price than U.S. manufacturers. After labor costs, health care is often the second largest supplier to many firms. In 1992, GM's health care expenses were about $1,500 per vehicle and were increasing faster than any other single cost incurred in the production of a vehicle. Unless health care costs can be controlled, so the executives claim, U.S. business will be priced out of international markets and foreign producers will increase their market share in the United States.

Do rising health costs really make U.S. industries less competitive than their foreign counterparts? To understand this controversy, it is important to understand who actually bears the burden of higher employee medical costs—the employee, the firm, or the consumer?

Who Pays for Higher Employee Medical Costs?

The market for labor is competitive. Large numbers of firms compete among themselves for different types of labor, and large numbers of employees compete for those jobs. This competition among firms and employees results in a price for labor that is similar for specific types of labor. For example, if a hospital pays its nurses less than other hospitals in the area, then its nurses will move to where the pay is highest. Not all nurses have to change jobs to bring about similar pay among hospitals. Some nurses will move, and the hospital will find it difficult to replace them. The hospital will soon realize that their pay levels are below what nurses are receiving elsewhere. In reality, not all firms have the same working conditions nor are they located next to one another. Employees are willing to accept lower pay for more pleasant conditions and require higher pay for traveling longer distances. The greater the similarity among firms in how they treat their employees and the more closely they are located to one another, the more quickly wage differences disappear.

When an employer hires an additional employee, the cost of that employee cannot exceed the value of that employee to the firm; otherwise, the firm will not find it profitable to hire the employee. The total cost to the firm of an employee consists of two parts: cash wages and noncash fringe benefits. The cost of hiring an additional worker is the total compensation, cash and noncash benefits, that the firm would have to pay to that employee. The employer does not care whether the employees want 90 percent of their total compensation in cash and 10 percent in noncash fringe benefits or a cash to noncash ratio of 60/40. The employer is only interested in the total cost of that employee.

Employees working in high-wage industries typically prefer a higher ratio of fringe benefits to cash wages because there are tax advantages to having benefits purchased with pretax income. Low-wage industries typically provide their employees with few benefits; most of their compensation is in cash income. The combination of cash and noncash income reflects the preferences of employees, not employers. If an employer compensated their low-wage employees with a high proportion of fringe benefits, the employees would seek the same total compensation at another firm that paid them a higher ratio of cash wages.

What happens when the fringe benefits portion of total compensation rises sharply, as occurs when health insurance premiums increase? For example, assume that employees in a particular industry are expected to receive a 5 percent increase in their compensation next year, and health insurance premiums, which are paid by the employer and represent 10 percent of the employees' total compensation, are expected to rise by 20 percent. The employer is always concerned with the total cost of its employees; thus cash wages in that industry would therefore rise by only 3.3 percent. There is a trade-off between fringe benefits and cash wages.

If one firm in the industry paid its employees 5 percent higher wages plus the 20 percent increase in insurance premiums, that firm would have higher labor costs than all the other firms in the industry. What are the consequences to the firm? To incur above-market labor costs, the firm would either have to make less profit or increase the prices of the products they sell. If they were to make less profit, they will earn a lower return on their invested capital. A lower return on invested capital will lead investors to move their capital to other firms in the industry, to other industries, or to other countries where they can earn a higher return. Capital knows no loyalties nor boundaries; it will move so as to receive the highest return (consistent with a given level of risk). Thus higher labor costs cannot impose a permanently lower return to a firm, otherwise the firm will shrink as it loses capital. The same would be true if labor costs among all firms in the industry increased and profits declined.

What if the firm or industry passed the higher labor costs on to consumers by raising its prices? As long as there are competitors to the firm's products, either from other firms in the industry or from manufacturers in other countries, and consumers are price sensitive to the firm's product, then the firm will lose sales. With lower sales, the firm will need fewer employees. There are generally good substitutes to any firm's (or industry's) product, either from other products or other manufacturers. Thus large price differences for the same or similar product cannot be maintained. The failure to keep prices in line with a competitor's prices will drastically reduce sales. The consequence would be a flight of capital from that firm or industry and a large reduction in the workforce.

As long as competition from other firms or from foreign competitors (or both) is possible and capital can move to other industries and countries, rising medical costs will not result in lower profits or higher prices but will be borne by employees in the form of lower cash wages.

Short-Term Effects

Even though rising medical costs are typically borne by the employee in the form of lower cash wages, it is possible that there could be a short-term effect on an employer's profits. It is difficult, in the short run, to shift the cost of health insurance back to employees. For example, if an employer did not anticipate how rapidly medical costs would increase and, perhaps because of a long-term labor agreement, the firm is unable to lower its employees' wages to compensate for the higher-than-expected medical costs, profitability could decline.

Few firms, however, are unaware of how rapidly medical costs are increasing. Thus rising costs are built into labor agreements. Medical costs could, however, also rise less rapidly than anticipated, thereby increasing profitability. In any case, unanticipated cost increases will be reflected in future wage agreements and would not affect profitability over time.

An Example

The following example illustrates why labor bears the burden of higher insurance premiums. Automobiles can be produced in Michigan or in the southern part of the U.S. Unless the prices of cars produced in Michigan and in the South are the same, consumers would purchase the least-expensive cars, assuming their quality is similar. And unless labor costs and productivity were similar in both places, the automobile manufacturers would move their production facilities to where it is less costly to produce the car. And yet we observe that within certain industries, such as automobiles, employees' medical costs and insurance premiums are higher in Detroit than they are for automobile employees in the South. How can cars produced in the North compete with cars produced in the South?

Medical costs per employee could be higher in the North as long as northern employees' cash wages are lower. Unless total compensation per employee is the same in both places, the cars produced in different locations could not be sold at the same price and manufacturers would shift their production to the lower-cost site.

The Effect of Unions

But what if an industry were strongly unionized and the firms in that industry were not permitted to hire nonunion labor. Could the union then shift its higher medical costs to the firm or to consumers? The extent to which a union can increase labor costs is always limited by the potential loss in its members' jobs. If U.S. manufacturers increase their prices relative to their competitors, foreign competition and price-sensitive consumers will cause them to suffer large declines in their sales and profits. Even when foreign competitors are prevented from competing with U.S. manufacturers, consumers would demand fewer automobiles as their price rises, although the declines would be less than if greater competition were permitted. Firms facing decreased demands for their products would hire fewer employees. A powerful union that is willing to accept a certain loss in its members' jobs by forcing firms to raise its members' compensation would do so regardless of whether it is for increased medical benefits or for higher wages. Thus increased medical benefits to the union members are still at the expense of higher wages.

Figure 17.1 illustrates the effect on employees' wages of rising medical costs. After 1973 total employee compensation rose less rapidly than previously because of a slowdown in employee productivity, and the difference between total compensation and wages increased as a greater portion of employees' total compensation went to pay for fringe benefits. Since 1973, employers' contributions to their employees' health insurance premiums "absorbed more than half of workers' real (adjusted for inflation) gains in compensation, even though health insurance represented 5 percent or less of total compensation" (Congressional Budget Office 1992, 5). Thus employees' wages over this period rose very slowly both because of low productivity growth and because most of the increase in compensation went to pay for higher health insurance premiums. Rising medical costs have therefore had a large effect on employees' take-home pay; they have had less to spend on other goods and services.

Who Pays for Retiree Medical Costs?

As part of their previous labor negotiations, many employers agreed to provide their employees with medical benefits when they retire in return for current wage concessions. Currently, about 40 percent of retirees between the ages of 65 and 69 are covered by their employer's retiree medical plan (Congressional Budget Office 1992, 39).[1] At the time employers agreed to provide their employees with medical benefits, retiree medical costs were much lower than they are today, and employers undoubtedly underestimated how costly they could become. And instead of setting aside funds to pay these retiree obligations, as one would do with a pension obligation, firms paid their retirees' medical costs on a "pay as you go" basis; that is, they paid their retirees' medical costs when they were incurred, out of current operating expenses.

Funding retiree medical costs changed as a result of a Financial Accounting Standards Board (FASB) rule, which stated that starting in 1993 firms must set aside funds for such benefits as they are earned.

Figure 17.1 Inflation-Adjusted Compensation and Wages per
Full-Time Employee, 1965–1992

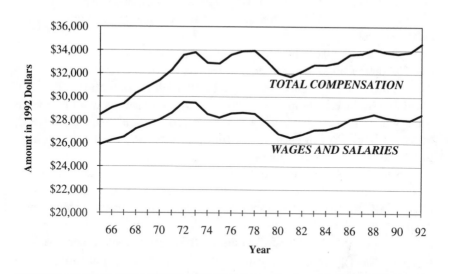

Note: Values adjusted for inflation using the consumer price index for all urban consumers.
Source: U.S. Department of Commerce, Bureau of Economic Analysis (Washington, DC).

Retiree medical benefits must be treated similarly to pension benefits. As employees earn credit toward their retirement, the firm must set aside funds to pay for that employee's medical costs when they retire. Further, the current unfunded liability for current and future retirees must be accounted for on the firm's balance sheet. Firms have been shocked by the size of their unfunded obligation. General Motors, for example, had to take a charge of $20 billion for their unfunded retirees' medical costs. As this liability is added to the balance sheet, an equivalent amount is deducted from the firm's net worth. General Motors stockholders' equity fell by $20 billion.

It has been estimated (in 1988) that these unfunded medical liabilities for both current and future retirees will reduce the net worth of corporations by $227 to $332 billion.

How are firms like General Motors going to pay off these huge unfunded liabilities? Will they raise the prices of their products, thereby harming U.S. competitiveness? They are unlikely to do so. If they were to raise their prices, they would lose sales to competitors, both in the United States and overseas, who have not made such commitments to their employees. Thus it is unlikely that U.S. competitiveness would be harmed by firms having to list unfunded retiree medical benefits on their balance sheet.

Employers also cannot reduce the wages of current employees to pay for their obligations to current retirees. If they were to do so, the firm would lose its employees. The labor market is competitive. If a firm decided to reduce its employees' wages, those employees would move to firms whose retirees have not been promised medical benefits. Instead, firms are likely to use current and future profits to pay off this liability, in which case the stockholders will be the losers.

Some firms are attempting to renege on their promise to their retirees by either reducing these benefits or by requiring retirees to pay part of the cost. Retirees have responded by bringing lawsuits against their former employers. The outcome of these lawsuits will determine whether firms are able to shift these obligations from their stockholders back to their retirees. Typically, only when a firm declares bankruptcy and is reorganized will it be able to reduce its obligations. If firms with large retiree liabilities declare bankruptcy, then the stockholders, bondholders, and retirees will all have to make some sacrifice for the firm to be viable again.

Rising medical costs will not directly affect U.S. competitiveness by forcing firms to increase their prices. Instead, these higher costs will be borne by the employees themselves who receive lower cash wages. The huge unfunded retiree medical liabilities will also not affect U.S. competitiveness because these liabilities will not be paid off by raising prices but will be shifted to the firm's stockholders in the form of reduced equity. Do rising medical costs then have any adverse effects on the economy and on U.S. competitiveness?

Possible Adverse Effects of Rising
Medical Costs on the U.S. Economy

Rising medical costs could adversely effect the U.S. balance of trade if they were to increase the federal deficit or if they decreased private savings.

Increase in the Federal Deficit

The argument on the deficit is as follows: government expenditures for Medicare and Medicaid are the fastest-increasing portion of the federal deficit. In 1970 federal spending on these two programs represented 1 percent of gross domestic product (GDP). By 1991 it had increased to 3 percent of GDP and is expected to reach 6.1 percent of GDP by 2002. If left unchanged, these two programs will represent 23 percent of the federal government's nonhealth spending by 2002 (Congressional Budget Office 1992, 7). To fund these additional expenditures, the government will have to increase its borrowing.

A higher level of government borrowing to finance a larger federal deficit will increase the value of the dollar relative to other currencies because interest rates in the United States will rise with the increased demand by government for savings and, in the process of moving their funds to the United States to take advantage of the higher interest rates, foreign investors will demand more dollars, which will increase their value. With a higher exchange value of the dollar, the prices of U.S. produced goods rise and foreign goods become less expensive. As the relative prices of U.S. and foreign goods change, domestic manufacturers will sell less overseas and imports will increase into this country as the price of foreign goods falls. American competitiveness and the trade balance will worsen.

There is, however, no reason to place the blame for the rising budget deficit on rising medical costs. Many government programs contribute to the deficit, and many are of less value than Medicare and Medicaid. The deficit could be reduced by reducing expenditures on these other programs as well, such as farm subsidies and military projects that have as their sole purpose maintaining jobs in a community. Emphasizing medical spending as the cause of the rising federal deficit shifts attention from these other government programs and reduces the government's incentives for eliminating wasteful government programs that provide less benefit than medical expenditures. It is also possible that reducing expenditures on Medicare and Medicaid would merely result in shifting these savings into expanding other, new government programs.

Reduction in Private Savings

The second way in which increased medical spending could adversely affect the American economy is if private savings were reduced. To finance the federal deficit, the government will have to borrow, which would leave less savings available for the private sector to invest in plant, equipment, and new ventures. Lower private investment eventually means lower productivity and lower real incomes. The Congressional

Budget Office estimates that if federal spending on Medicare and Medicaid were limited to its 1991 share of the gross domestic product, real incomes could be 2.4 percent higher by the year 2002.

Similarly to the above, rising medical costs cause the public to spend more on medical services, thereby decreasing the amount it has available to save. As a consequence, savings in the private sector decline and with it a decrease in private investment.

The argument blaming the lower rate of savings on rising medical expenditures is similar to blaming the federal deficit on Medicare and Medicaid. The government could reduce the deficit by eliminating and reducing other government programs. Medicare and Medicaid are not the sole cause for large federal deficits.

It is not clear that rising medical costs decrease or increase the private savings rate. Having health insurance may reduce the need for a person to save for their medical expenses. However, medical expenses increase with age, there are increasing out-of-pocket payments that may be required, and as people live longer they will have to save for their long-term care needs if they do not want to rely on Medicaid (and have to spend down their assets to qualify). The expectation of higher medical costs and new technology may cause people to increase their savings. The effect of rising medical expenses on savings is uncertain.

There is also a fallacy that the rise in medical expenditures should be limited because it increases consumption, thereby reducing savings for investment. Some medical expenditures are in fact investments that increase productivity, such as preventive measures and certain surgical procedures that enable a person to resume normal activity. But more importantly, if it is desired to increase the savings rate by decreasing consumption, there are many other consumer activities, some of which are harmful, such as alcohol and cigarette consumption, that should probably be reduced before limits are placed on medical spending. Many people would place a higher value on medical services than on other goods and services.

Summary

Thus it is not clear that increased medical spending has harmful effects on the economy, on the budget deficit, or on American competitiveness, as some would suggest.

The fact that employees rather than employers bear the cost of rising health care benefits should, however, not mean that employers are absolved from the responsibility of ensuring that those funds are well spent. As Uwe Reinhardt stated,

> Even if every increase in the cost of employer-paid health care benefits could immediately be financed by the firm with commensurate reductions in the cash compensation of its employees—so that "competitiveness" in the firm's product market is not impaired—it would leave employees worse off unless the added health spending is valued at least as highly as the cash wages they would forego [sic] to finance these benefits. Because it is the perceived value of a firm's compensation package that lures workers to the firm and away from competing opportunities, the typical business firm has every economic incentive to maximize this perceived value per dollar of health care expenditure debited to the firm's payroll expense account. Therein, and not in "competitiveness" on the product side, lies the most powerful rationale for vigorous health care cost containment on the part of the American business community (1989, 20).

Note

1. Early retirees who are not eligible for Medicare are more costly than those who are. For retirees on Medicare, the firm usually pays for that portion of the retirees' medical expense not covered by Medicare, such as deductibles, copayments, and prescription drugs.

References

Reinhardt, U. E. "Health Care Spending and American Competitiveness." *Health Affairs* 8 (Winter 1989): 20.

U.S. Congressional Budget Office. *Economic Implications of Rising Health Care Costs*. Washington, DC: Congressional Budget Office, 1992.

18

Why Is It So Difficult to Get into Medical School?

In 1991, only 17,000 of the 33,300 students who applied to 126 medical schools in the United States were accepted, for an applicant to acceptance ratio of 1.95:1. The ratio, having reached a high of 2.8:1 in 1973, steadily declined to 1.58:1 in 1988 but now has started to rise again. As shown in Figure 18.1, first-year medical school enrollments increased sharply in the late 1960s mostly because federal legislation (The Health Manpower Training Act of 1964) gave medical schools strong financial incentives to increase their enrollments. When these federal subsidies phased out, enrollments leveled out and have remained relatively steady since the early 1980s. There remains, however, a continual excess demand for a medical education.

Many qualified students are rejected each year because of the limited number of medical school spaces. Some rejected students choose to enroll in medical schools in other countries, such as Mexico. Overseas medical schools often charge higher tuition and require longer training periods than U.S. medical schools, which require four years of college prior to receiving four years of medical school. Residency training then requires an additional three to seven years of graduate medical education. Unfortunately, medical education is one area where academic excellence is not a sufficient qualification for admission to graduate or professional education. Other types of graduate-level professional education programs have experienced sharp increases in demand but not continual excess demands for admission. Although every well-qualified student who wants

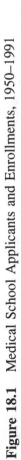

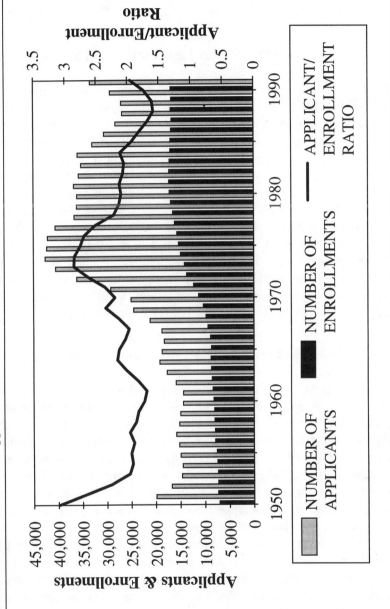

Figure 18.1 Medical School Applicants and Enrollments, 1950–1991

Sources: American Association of Medical Colleges (Washington, DC), *Medical School Admission Requirements*, various editions.

to become a physicist, mathematician, economist, or lawyer cannot re-alistically expect to be admitted to his or her first choice in graduate schools, if such students have good academic qualifications, as do most medical students, they will be admitted to some U.S. graduate school.[1]

The Market for Medical Education in Theory

When medicine is perceived as being relatively more attractive than other careers, demand for medical schools will increase and exceed the available number of spaces; a shortage of medical school spaces will occur. If the market for medical education were like other markets, this shortage would only be temporary while more medical schools are being built and existing schools recruit additional faculty and add physicial facilities to meet the increased demand. Over time the temporary short-age would be resolved as the supply of spaces is increased. Crucial in eliminating a temporary shortage is a rise in price (tuition). Increased tuition would serve to ration student demand among the existing number of spaces and would provide medical schools with a financial incentive (and the funds) to invest in facilities and faculty so they can accommodate larger enrollments. Subsidies and loan programs could be made available directly to low-income students faced with higher tuition rates.

The Market for Medical Education in Practice

The market for medical education, however, differs from other markets. The medical education industry produces its output inefficiently (at high cost and using too many years of the student's time), it produces the wrong type of output (too many specialists and not enough primary care physicians), and the method used to finance medical education is inequitable (large subsidies go to students from high-income families). Any other industry with this record would have been driven out of business by more efficient competitors. How has this industry been able to survive with such poor performance?

The producers of medical education have been insulated from the marketplace. Tuition, established at an arbitrarily low level, represents less than one-third of the costs of education and approximately 10 percent of medical school revenues. Medical schools can maintain low tuition because large state subsidies and research grants offset educational costs. Tuition, being such a small fraction of educational costs and not rising with increased demand, neither serves to ration excess demand among students nor provides an incentive to medical schools to expand their capacity. Medical schools, particularly public ones, do not depend upon tuition revenue to even cover their operating expenses.

Lacking a financial incentive to expand, medical schools do nothing to alleviate the temporary shortage. Instead, the shortage becomes permanent, which is far more serious.

For-profit businesses respond to increased consumer demands both by raising their prices and by increasing supplies because they want to make greater profits. New firms enter industries where they perceive they can earn more on their investment than they can earn elsewhere. When prices are prevented from rising or there are barriers to new firms entering an expanding market, temporary shortages can become permanent. Typically, barriers to entry are legal rather than economic and protect existing firms from competition. Protected firms are able to maintain higher prices and receive above-normal profits than if new firms were permitted to enter the market.

Medical schools, being not-for-profit organizations, are motivated by more "noble" goals, such as the "prestige" associated with training tomorrow's medical educators. Most medical schools share the goal of having a renowned, research-oriented faculty who teach a few small classes of academically gifted students, who will be their successors as superspecialist researchers. Few, if any, medical schools seek acclaim for graduating large numbers of primary care physicians who practice in underserved areas.

Only by maintaining an excess demand for admissions can medical schools choose the type of student who will become the type of physician they prefer (who will meet their prestige goals). Both the type of student selected and the design of the educational curriculum are determined by the desires of the medical school faculty, not by what is needed to train quality physicians efficiently (in terms of both student time and cost per student). As long as there is a permanent shortage of medical school spaces, medical schools will continue to "profit" by selecting the type of student the faculty desires, establishing educational requirements the faculty deems most appropriate, and producing graduates who mirror the faculty's preferences. Thus it is that the current system of medical education contains inadequate incentives for medical schools to respond, cost-effectively, to changes in the demand for medical education.

How likely is it that a large, managed care organization could start its own self-supporting medical school, one that would admit students after only two years of undergraduate training (as is done in Great Britain), with a revised curriculum and residency requirement that would combine the last two years of medical school with the first two years of graduate medical education, thereby reducing the graduate medical education requirement by one year (as proposed by the former dean of the Harvard Medical School), and financed either by tuition or by their graduates repaying their tuition by practicing for a number of years in their organization? Such schools could satisfy the excess demands for a medical education, reduce the educational process by at least three years, and, at the same time, teach students to be practitioners in a managed care environment (Ebert and Ginzberg 1988).

Accreditation for Medical Schools

Not surprisingly, starting new and innovative medical schools is very difficult. The Liaison Committee on Medical Education (LCME) accredits programs leading to the MD degree and establishes the criteria to which a school must adhere if it is to be accredited (Association of American Medical Colleges and the American Medical Association 1991). For example, a minimum number of weeks of instruction and calendar years (four) for the instruction to occur are specified, and an undergraduate education, usually four years, is required for admission to a medical school. Innovations in curriculum and changes in the length of time for becoming a physician (and to prepare for admission to medical school) must be approved by the LCME. The LCME further states that the cost of a medical education should be supported from diverse sources: tuition, endowment, faculty earnings, government grants and appropriations, parent university, and gifts. By its concern that there should not be too great a reliance on tuition, the LCME encourages the schools to pursue revenue sources and goals unrelated to educational concerns.

To be accredited, medical schools must also be not-for-profit. The LCME's accreditation criteria eliminate, in effect, all incentives for HMOs and similar organizations to invest in medical schools in hopes of earning a profit or having a steady supply of practitioners. There is no incentive for private organizations to invest capital to start a new school.

The status quo of the current high-cost medical education system would be threatened if graduates of these new medical schools proved as qualified as those trained in more traditional schools (as evidenced by their licensure examination scores and by their performance in residencies offered to them) and could enter practice three years earlier.

Instead, to bring about medical education reform there have been nine commissions since the 1960s to recommend changes. In a 1989 survey, medical school deans, department chairs, and faculty overwhelmingly endorsed the need for "fundamental changes" or "thorough reform" in medical student education. One examination of the lack of medical education reform indicated that

> faculty lack sufficient incentives to participate in the reform of medical education programs, because promotion and tenure are based primarily on research productivity and clinical practice expertise . . . [there is] the relegation of students' education to a secondary position within the medical school . . . Faculty have tended to think of the goals of their own academic specialty and department rather than the educational goals of the school as a whole (Enarson and Burg 1992).

Recommended Changes

It is not surprising that without financial incentives, a not-for-profit sector will fail to respond to increased student demands for a medical education and will not be concerned with the efficiency by which medical education is provided. Instead of relying on innumerable commissions whose proposed reforms go largely unimplemented, three changes in the current system of medical education and quality assurance should be considered: (1) ease the entry requirements for starting new medical schools, (2) reduce medical school subsidies, and (3) place more emphasis on monitoring physician practice patterns.

Ease the Entry Requirements for Starting New Medical Schools

The accreditation criteria of the LCME should be changed to permit managed care organizations (including those that are for-profit) to start medical schools. A larger number of schools competing for students would pressure medical schools to be more innovative and efficient. With easier entry into the medical education market, it will be necessary to shift the emphasis on quality from the process of becoming a physician toward quality outcomes, namely, toward examinations and the monitoring of physicians' practice behavior. Directly monitoring physicians' practice behavior is the most effective way for protecting the public against unethical and incompetent physicians.

As more physicians participate in managed care organizations and in large medical groups associated with these organizations, physician peer review will be enhanced. These organizations have a financial incentive to evaluate the quality and appropriateness of care given by physicians under their auspices since these organizations compete with similar organizations according to their premiums, the quality of care provided, and access to services. Quality assurance of physician services will increase as a result of competition among these large organizations.

Reduce Medical School Subsidies

In addition to relaxing the entry barriers to providing medical education, reducing government subsidies would cause medical schools to become more efficient by reducing the time required for a medical degree and the costs of providing it. There is no reason why medical students should be subsidized to a greater extent than students in other graduate or professional schools. A decrease in state subsidies to medical schools will force medical schools to reexamine and reduce their costs of education. Medical schools that merely raise their tuition to make up the lost revenues will find it difficult to attract a sufficient number of highly qualified applicants, once there are more schools competing for students. As tuition more accurately reflects the cost of education, applicants will comparison shop and evaluate schools with a range of tuition levels. To be competitive, schools with a lesser reputation will have to have corresponding lower tuition levels. The need to reduce student educational costs most likely will result in innovative curriculums, new teaching methods, and better use of the medical student's time.

To assure that every qualified student has an equal opportunity to become a physician once subsidies are decreased, student loan and subsidy programs must be made available. Current low tuition rates subsidize, in effect, the medical education of all medical students, even those who come from high-income families. And once these students graduate, they enter one of the highest-income professions. It would be more equitable to provide subsidies directly to qualified students according to their family income levels. Providing the subsidies directly to the students in the form of a voucher (to be used only in a medical school) would be an incentive for students to select a medical school according to its reputation, the total costs of education, and the number of years of education required to graduate (college and medical school). Medical schools would be forced to compete for students according to cost, years of training, and reputation.

Place More Emphasis on Monitoring Physician Practice Patterns

Currently, the process for ensuring physician quality relies wholly on graduation from an approved medical school and the passing of a licensing examination. Once a physician is licensed, no reexamination is required to maintain that license (although specialty boards may impose their own requirements for admission and maintenance of membership). State licensing boards are responsible for monitoring physicians' behavior and for penalizing physicians whose performance is inadequate or whose conduct is unethical. Unfortunately, this approach for assuring physician quality and competence is completely inadequate.

State licensing boards discipline very few physicians. In 1969, not even one in a thousand physicians (.69 per 1,000 physicians) received any disciplinary action. Between 1980 and 1982, the disciplinary rate rose slightly—to 1.3 per 1,000 physicians, or one-tenth of one percent of all physicians. Recently, a change in the reporting of disciplinary actions, which increased the base number, has made it difficult to compare with previous numbers. But, in 1991 in the United States, the "total number of prejudicial acts (PAs) per 1,000 practicing in-state physicians" was 4.79, or one-half of one percent of all physicians. Disciplinary actions vary greatly by state. Some states take virtually no disciplinary actions against their physicians. The number of PAs per 1,000 physicians in large states varied from a low of 1.21 in Pennsylvania to a high of 12.47 in Florida. The number of PAs per 1,000 physicians in other large states was 1.63 in New York, 5.28 in New Jersey, and 2.9 in California (*Journal of the American Medical Association* 1992).

It is unlikely that Florida has more unethical or incompetent physicians than other states. Instead, the considerable variability from state to state represents the uneven efforts by the medical licensing boards of those states, who are mainly physicians, to monitor and discipline physicians in their states. In fact, even when physicians lose their license in one state, they can move to another state and practice there; some state medical boards encourage physicians to move to another state in exchange for dropping charges. Only 14 states (as of 1991) permit their licensing boards to act based solely on another state's findings. The public is not as protected from incompetent and unethical medical practitioners as they have been led to believe.

Monitoring the care provided by physicians through the use of claims and medical records data would more directly determine the quality and competence of a physician. State licensing boards need to devote more resources to monitoring physician behavior. Also, requiring periodic reexamination and relicensing of all physicians would make physicians update their skills and knowledge. Rather than requiring physicians to take a minimum number of hours of continuing education, reexamination would determine the appropriate amount of continuing education on an individual basis. (Continuing education by itself is a "process" measure for ensuring quality and does not ensure that physicians actually maintain and update their skills and knowledge base.) Reexamination is a more useful and direct measure for assessing whether a physician has achieved the objectives of continuing education.

Periodic reexamination and relicensure would determine what tasks an individual physician is proficient enough to perform. Currently, all licensed physicians are permitted to perform a wide range of tasks, even though for some they may have insufficient training. Physicians may designate themselves as specialists whether or not they are certified by a specialty board. Legally, at present, any physician can perform surgery, provide anesthesia services, and diagnose patients. Reexamination could result in a physician's practice being limited to those tasks for which he or she continues to demonstrate proficiency. Instead of "all or nothing" licenses, physicians would be granted specific-purpose licenses. Such a licensing process would acknowledge that licensing physicians to perform a wide range of medical tasks does not serve the best interests of the public because not all physicians are qualified to perform all tasks adequately.

Specific-purpose licensure would mean that not all physicians would need to take the same educational training; training in some specialties would take a much shorter period of time, while training to become a superspecialist would, of course, take longer. Shorter educational requirements for family practitioners would both lower the cost of their medical education and enable them to graduate earlier, thereby earning an income sooner. Even with higher tuition, family practitioners would incur a smaller debt and could begin paying it off at least three years earlier. The number of family practitioners would increase since they would have to make a much smaller investment (fewer years of both schooling and lost income) in their medical education, which would more than compensate for not receiving as high an income as a specialist. When a physician wants an additional specific-purpose license, he or she could receive additional training and then take the qualifying exam for that license. The training requirements for entering the medical profession would be determined not by the medical profession, but by the demand for different types of physicians and the least-cost manner of producing them.

Summary

The competition among medical schools that would result from reducing their subsidies and permitting new schools to enter would improve the performance of the market for medical education. Easing entry restrictions would make it easier for nontraditional schools to be started (and for existing schools to innovate), thereby making it easier for qualified students to be admitted to a medical school. Qualified students would no longer have to incur the higher expense and longer training times of attending a foreign medical school. Emphasizing outcome measures and appropriateness of care will better protect the public from incompetent and unethical physicians. Reduction of government subsidies to medical schools would force medical schools to be more efficient and innovative in structuring and producing a medical education. And distributing subsidies to students according to their family income rather than to the medical school (which results in a subsidy to all students) would enhance equity among students receiving a medical education.

Note

1. Medical education also differs from other graduate programs in that once accepted to medical school, the student is virtually assured of graduating. The attrition rate is approximately 3 percent compared to attrition rates of 50 percent in other graduate programs.

References

Association of American Medical Colleges and the American Medical Association. *Liaison Committee on Medical Education, Functions and Structure of a Medical School.* Washington, DC: Association of American Medical Colleges and the American Medical Association, 1991.

Ebert, R. H., and E. Ginzberg. "The Reform of Medical Education." *Health Affairs* 7 (Supplement 1988): 5–38.

Enarson, C., and F. Burg. "An Overview of Reform Initiatives in Medical Education: 1906 through 1992." *Journal of the American Medical Association* 268 (2 September 1992): 1141–43.

Journal of the American Medical Association "From the Federation of State Medical Boards of the United States." 267 (3 June 1992): 2857–59.

19

The Shortage of Nurses

Throughout the post–World War II period, there have been recurrent concerns over a national shortage of registered nurses (RNs). At times the shortage of nurses seemed particularly acute; at other times it appeared to be resolved, only to reassert itself several years later. Government and private commissions have attempted to quantify the magnitude of the shortage and have proposed remedies. The federal government has, since 1964, spent billions of dollars to alleviate the nursing shortage. Given the continuing concern over the shortage of nurses and the large federal subsidies that have gone to support nursing education, it is useful to examine why there is a shortage of nurses and what, if anything, should be done about it.

Measuring Nursing Shortages

The measure commonly used to indicate a shortage of nurses is the nurse vacancy rate in hospitals—the percent of unfilled nursing positions for which hospitals are recruiting. The vacancy rate was at a high of 23 percent in 1962, steadily declined throughout the 1960s, and reached single digits by the early 1970s; it rose in the late 1970s, reaching 14 percent in 1979, but by 1983 fell to 4.4 percent. By the mid-1980s, the vacancy rate was climbing again and exceeded 12 percent by 1989, after which it declined to 5.3 percent in 1992 (for vacancy rates from 1979 to 1992, see Figure 19.1).

Figure 19.1   RN Vacancy Rates, 1979–1992

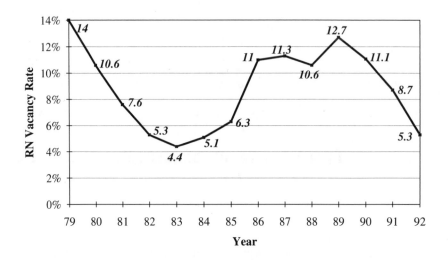

Sources: American Hospital Association, Division of Nursing and the Hospital Data Center (Chicago, IL), *Report of the Hospital Nursing Personnel Survey*, various editions.

Each of these periods of high or rising registered nurse vacancy rates brought forth commissions to study the problem and make recommendations. The high vacancy rates in the early 1960s led to the start of federal support for nursing education, the Nurse Training Act of 1964, which has been renewed many times since then.

Nursing Shortages in Theory

What are the reasons for a shortage of registered nurses? The definition of a nurse shortage is that hospitals cannot hire all the nurses they want *at the current wage*. In other words, at the existing wage, the demand for nurses exceeds the number of nurses willing to work at that wage. However, economic theory claims that if the demand for nurses exceeds the supply of nurses, hospitals will compete among themselves for nurses, and nurses' wages would increase. As nurses' wages rise, nurses who are not working will seek employment; part-time nurses will be willing to increase the hours they work. All those hospitals willing to pay the new, higher wage will be able to hire all the nurses they want. Hospitals would no longer have vacancies for nurses.

Economic theory would thus predict that if there are shortages, we would expect to observe rising wages for nurses followed by declining vacancy rates. Nurse employment will increase (more nurses enter the labor force and others work longer hours), and as nurses' wages increase, hospitals will not hire as many nurses at the higher wage as they initially wanted. Shortages could recur if the demand for nurses once again increases. With an increase in demand, the process starts over; hospitals find they cannot hire all they want at the current wage, and so on. Clearly, wages are not the only reason why nurses work or why they increase their hours of work. The nurse's age, whether or not he or she has young children, and overall family income are also important considerations. A change in the nurse's wage, however, will affect the benefits of working versus not working and thereby affect the nurse's choice of hours worked.

Nursing Shortages in Practice

How well does economic theory that relies on increased demand for nurses explain the recurrent shortages of nurses? It is important to separate nurse shortages into two time periods, the periods before and after the 1965 passage of Medicare and Medicaid.

Before the Passage of Medicare and Medicaid

Before Medicare, the vacancy rate kept rising, exceeding 20 percent by the early 1960s. Hospital demand for nurses continued to exceed the supply of nurses at a given wage. Surprisingly, however, nurses' wages did not rise as rapidly as wages in comparable occupations, which were not even subject to the same shortage pressures. Over a period of years, worsening shortages of nurses and limited rises in nurse wages could only have been the result of interference with the process by which wages were determined.

Working on the hypothesis that nurse wages were being artificially held down, economist Donald Yett found that hospitals were colluding among themselves to prevent nurses' wages from rising. The hospitals believed that competing among themselves for nurses would merely result in large nurse wage increases (hence a large increase in hospital costs) without bringing forth a large increase in the number of employed nurses. This collusive behavior by hospitals on the setting of nurses' wages prevented the shortage from being resolved. (For additional references on the nursing shortage and a more complete discussion of the shortage over time, see Feldstein 1993.)

After the Passage of Medicare and Medicaid

Once Medicare and Medicaid were enacted, hospitals were reimbursed according to their costs for treating Medicare and Medicaid patients. Consequently, hospitals were more willing to increase nurse wages. Nurses' wages increased rapidly in the mid- to late 1960s and the vacancy rate declined from 23 percent in 1962 to 9.3 percent by 1971. The increase in nurses' wages brought about a large increase in the number of employed nurses, contrary to hospitals' earlier expectations. The number of nonworking (trained) nurses that decided to reenter nursing rose, from 55 percent in 1960, to 65 percent in 1966, to 70 percent in 1972. Increased wages had an important effect on nurse participation rates.

The artificial shortages created by hospitals before the mid-1960s are no longer possible. The antitrust laws make it illegal for hospitals to collude to hold down nurses' wages. The recurrent shortage of nurses since that time has been of a different type.

The lack of information in the market for nurses lengthens the time necessary to resolve shortages. For example, if a hospital experiences an increase in its admissions, it will try and hire more nurses. The hospital may, however, find that its personnel department cannot hire more nurses at the going wage. The hospital's vacancy rate increases. Other hospitals in the community may have the same experience. The hospital then has to decide whether and by how much to raise the wage of nurses to attract additional nurses. If the hospital decides to raise nurses' wages, it will have to pay the higher wage to its existing nurses as well. The hospital must then decide, at the higher wage for new nurses and for all its existing nurses, how many additional nurses it can afford to hire. The cost of a new nurse is not only the wage they must pay that new nurse but also the cost of increasing wages to all the other nurses as well.

The hospital may decide that rather than increasing wages, it is less costly to try other approaches for recruiting new nurses, such as providing child care and a more supportive environment. There is thus a time lag between the period when the hospital decides to hire more nurses, raising wages, and being satisfied with the number of nurses it has.

There is also a time lag before the supply of nurses responds to changed market conditions. Once nurses' wages are increased, it takes time for this information to become widely disseminated. Nurses who are not working may decide to return to nursing at the higher wage; this would be indicated by an increase in the nurse participation rate. Other nurses who are working part-time may decide to increase the number of hours they work, and with higher wages, more high school graduates may decide to undertake the educational requirements to become a nurse. The most rapid response to an increase in wages will come from those who are part-time and then from those who are already trained but not working as a nurse. The long-run supply of nurses is determined by those who decide to enter nursing schools. There are thus short- and long-run supply responses to an increase in nurses' wages.

Let us now return to an examination of how well economic theory explains the recurrent shortage of nurses. Throughout the late 1960s and early 1970s, nurses' wages increased more rapidly than wages in comparable professions, such as teachers. The result was declining vacancy rates and increased participation of nurses. However, by the late 1970s there were concerns of a new shortage of nurses. In 1979 the vacancy rate reached 14 percent. The shortage was, however, short-lived. Nurses' wages rose sharply and a recession in the general economy occurred in the early 1980s.

The rising unemployment rate caused more nurses to seek employment and to increase their hours of work. Seventy percent of RNs are married, and their spouse's income is an important part of total family income. The loss of a job by a spouse, or even the fear of losing a job, is likely to cause nurses to increase their labor force participation to maintain their family incomes (Buerhaus 1993).

The effect of higher wages and the rising unemployment rate resulted in an increase in the nurse participation rate from 70 percent in 1972 to 76 percent in 1980 and 79 percent in 1984. Vacancy rates dropped to 4.4 percent by 1983. The nursing shortage was once again resolved through a combination of rising wages, an increase in the nurse participation rate, and the national unemployment rate.

In the 1980s the market for hospital services underwent drastic changes, which in turn affected the market for nurses. The trend by both government and private insurers to reduce use of the hospital resulted in shorter hospital lengths of stay. This meant that patients required more intensive treatment for the shorter time they were in the hospital. As a result, hospitals increased their use of registered nurses to provide more intensive care for the patients. The recovery period, which requires less intensive care, was occurring outside the hospital.

Changes in the organization of hospital nursing units were also occurring during this period. Registered nurses were able to be used more flexibly than licensed practical nurses (because of their training and state practice acts) in performing tasks on a nursing unit. Nursing units moved toward using a greater proportion of (or even all) registered nurses in their staffing patterns. Registered nurses as a proportion of all nursing personnel rose from 33 percent in 1968 to 46 percent in 1980 to 65 percent by 1990.

Indicative of hospitals' increased demand for nurses because of changes in staffing patterns and patients needing more intensive care is the trend in the number of registered nurses per patient in community hospitals. In 1975 there were .65 RNs per patient; it climbed to .88 in 1980, and to 1.34 RNs per patient by 1990.

There was also an increase in the demand for nurses in outpatient and nonhospital settings. As the use of the hospital declined, use of outpatient care, nursing homes, home care, and hospices for terminally ill Medicare patients increased. Between 1980 and 1991, outpatient visits increased from 262 million to almost 400 million visits, use by Medicare patients of skilled nursing homes increased from 8,645 to 24,126 days, home health visits increased from 16,322 to 77,970, and hospice admissions increased from 2,200 (in 1984 when it became a Medicare benefit) to 112,595 (Prospective Payment Assessment Commission 1992). In addition to providing care in these alternative settings, there was an increased demand for registered nurses by cost-containment companies to conduct utilization review and case management.

As the demand for nurses in all these different settings increased faster than supply in the mid- to late 1980s, nurses' wages were slow to respond, and the national unemployment rate declined (see Figure 19.2). As a consequence, vacancy rates once again began to rise, reaching 12.7 percent in 1989. By the late 1980s there was again concern over a shortage of nurses.

Economic incentives, however, are once again causing that shortage to disappear. At the beginning of the 1990s a recession started and unemployment began to rise. The supply of nurses increased. The nurse participation rate (both full- and part-time employed nurses) reached 80 percent (the participation rate for all women is only 54 percent). By 1990 the vacancy rate declined to 11 percent and then fell to 5.3 percent in 1992.

Since the mid-1960s, the recurrent shortages of nurses have been caused by increased demands for nurses and the failure by hospitals to

Figure 19.2 RN Vacancy Rates, Annual Percent Changes in Real
RN Wages, and the National Unemployment Rate,
1979–1992

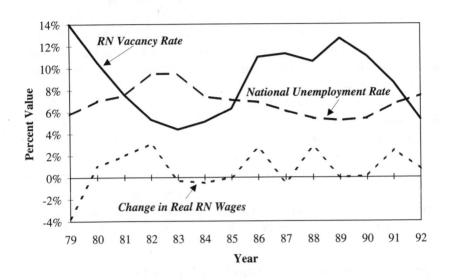

Source: Reprinted with permission, as it appeared in Peter I. Buerhaus, "Capitalizing on the Recession's Effect on Hospital RN Shortages," *Hospital & Health Services Administration* 39, no. 1 (Spring): 51. © Foundation of the American College of Healthcare Executives, 1994.

immediately recognize that, at the higher demand, nurses' wages must be increased. Once hospitals realize that the market conditions for nurses has changed, the process starts that once again brings equilibrium to the market. It appears to take several years before equilibrium is again achieved. Higher wages reduce the number of nurses demanded by hospitals, part-time nurses increase their hours of work, and the participation of nurses increases. These are the typical elements of the adjustment process. At times the start of a recession, as occurred at the beginning of the 1980s and 1990s, has increased the supply of nurses still further, thereby shortening the time for the shortage to be resolved.

Nursing School Enrollments

Increases in nurses' wages to resolve shortages also affect the future supply of nurses. As nurses' wages have risen faster than those in comparable occupations, more high school graduates have chosen a nursing career. There is always a lag of several years before the information on nurses' wages is transmitted to high school graduates and nursing school enrollments change. The sharp increase in nurses' wages after the passage of Medicare in the mid-1960s led to a rapid increase in nursing school enrollments (see Figure 19.3). When nurse wage increases slowed in the late 1970s, nursing school enrollments fell. As nurse vacancy rates increased in the late 1970s and nurses' wages increased, enrollments rose by the early 1980s.

Declining nurse enrollments in the latter half of the 1980s reflected the slow growth in nurse wages, a declining nurse vacancy rate, and two changes affecting our entire society: changing age demographics and expanded career opportunities for women. Demographics have reduced the number of high school graduates that are eligible for a nursing career. More importantly, the larger number of career opportunities open to women in the 1980s, such as in teaching, business, and medicine, led to a reduction in the percent of college-age women choosing a nursing career.

Figure 19.3   Nursing School Enrollments, 1960–1991

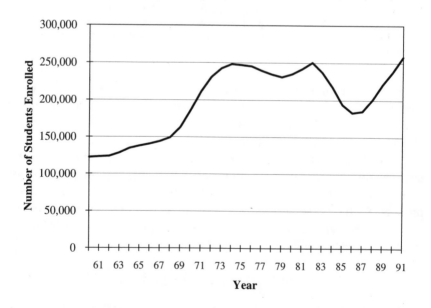

Sources: American Nurses Association, *Facts about Nursing*, various editions.

Even with these broader societal trends, market forces continue to affect the future supply of nurses. Enrollment in nursing schools began to again increase in 1988, two years after nurse wages and the nurse vacancy rate began their increase (see Figure 19.2). This upward trend in nursing school enrollments became stronger and continued into the early 1990s, reflecting the previous growth in demand for nurses. Given the current downward trend in "real" nurse wages and vacancy rates, as shown in Figure 19.2, it would not be surprising to observe a new decline in nursing school enrollments.

Federal Subsidies to Nursing Schools and Students

High vacancy rates, demographic trends, alternative career opportunities for women, and the already high nurse participation rate have led to calls for increased federal subsidies to nursing schools and for student loans to increase the supply of nurses. Proposals for federal funding to increase the supply of nurses have been made since the enactment of the 1964 Nurse Training Act and its many renewals. These recommendations ignore the important role played by higher wages in increasing both the short- and long-run supply of nurses. The adjustment process is relatively quick.

Federal subsidies to nursing schools and students cannot be directed only to those students who would otherwise have chosen a different career. Nurse education subsidies take years before they have an effect on the supply of nurses. More importantly, to the extent that federal programs are successful in increasing the number of nursing school graduates, nurses' wages would rise more slowly. A larger supply of new graduates would cause a lower rate of increase in nurses' wages, which in turn would result in a smaller increase in the nurse participation rate. Nurses would be more reluctant to return to nursing or to increase their hours of work if their wages did not increase.

Reliance on market mechanisms rather than on federal subsidies to solve nurse shortages is likely to bring about a quicker resolution of that shortage. First, future demand increases for nurses can be met by increasing the number of hours that part-time nurses work. One-third of all employed nurses, more than 600,000, work part-time. Increased wages that induce these nurses to increase their hours of work can result in large increases in the supply of nursing time. Second, higher wages for nurses will cause hospitals and other demanders of nurses to rethink how they use their nurses. As nurses become more expensive to employ, hospitals will use nurses in higher-skilled tasks and delegate to lesser-trained nursing personnel, such as licensed practical nurses, certain housekeeping and other tasks currently performed by registered nurses. It has been estimated that up to 50 percent of nurses' time is spent on tasks that can be delegated to others. Third, higher wages and new roles for nurses will make nursing a more attractive profession. Lastly, nursing has been a female profession. There is no reason why more males cannot be attracted to a nursing career. Higher wages and new nursing roles will increase the attractiveness of nursing to a larger segment of the population.

The Future of Nursing

The potential supply of nurses is not as limited as many believe. To realize the full potential of nursing as a profession and to expand the supply of nurses, more information must be provided to both the demanders and suppliers in this market. Demanders must be made more aware of approaches that increase nurses' productivity and the wages and other working conditions necessary to attract more nurses. Nurses, particularly those who are not employed or who are working part-time, have to be aware of opportunities in nursing, as well as wages and working conditions being offered. High school students need information if they are to make informed career choices. Efforts to increase information are more likely to eliminate shortages and lead to an increase in the supply of nurses than policies that instead merely rely on large federal subsidies to nursing education.

The nursing profession faces both challenges and opportunities in coming years. Both public policy and private initiatives are directed at reducing the rising cost of medical care. If the outcome of public policy is arbitrary budget limits on hospitals and on total medical expenditures, nurses' wages will not increase as rapidly as wages for comparably trained professions in the nonregulated health sector. Innovation in the use of RNs and in the provision of new medical services will be stifled for lack of funds.

If, however, public policy reinforces what is occurring in the private sector, namely, competition among managed care organizations on the basis of their premiums and quality of care, the demand for registered nurses will be determined by their productivity, the tasks they are permitted to perform, and their wages, relative to other types of nursing personnel. To the extent that RNs are more costly than LPNs for similar tasks, these organizations will shift toward greater use of LPNs. However, to the extent that RNs are able to perform more highly valued tasks, such as assuming responsibility for more primary care services (given the shortage of primary care physicians), utilization review services, and managing home health care, as is currently the case in many competitive areas, they become more valuable to managed care organizations, who would be willing to increase their use of RNs and their wages to reflect the higher value of services rendered.

The future roles, responsibilities, and incomes of registered nurses will be very much affected by the direction that health care reform takes in coming years.

References

Buerhaus, P. I. "Effects of RN Wages and Non-Wage Income on the Performance of the Hospital RN Labor Market." *Nursing Economic$*, 11 (June 1993): 129–34.

Feldstein, P. J. *Health Care Economics*, 4th ed. Albany, NY: Delmar Publishers, 1993. (See Chapter 16, "The Market for Registered Nurses.")

Prospective Payment Assessment Commission. *Medicare and the American Health Care System: Report to the Congress*. Washington, DC: Prospective Payment Assessment Commission, 1992.

20

The High Price of Prescription Drugs

Since the early 1980s, prices for prescription drugs have been rising much more rapidly than the consumer price index, as shown in Figure 20.1. Insurance coverage for prescription drugs, while slowly increasing over time, remains low. As shown in Figure 20.2, patients pay a higher percent (55 percent) of drug expenditures out-of-pocket than they do for any other major health expenditure. Paying for high-priced prescription drugs is a hardship for many AIDS victims and for the aged on fixed incomes, and rising drug expenditures are becoming an increasing burden to state Medicaid programs. Yet, pharmaceutical company profits continue to be among the highest of any industry.

This chapter addresses two issues: Why are drug prices rising so rapidly? And is public policy needed to lower drug prices?

Reasons for Rising Drug Prices

Prices could rise for several reasons: the cost of producing the product could increase, the demand conditions facing the producer could change, or an improved version of the product comes on the market at a higher price. Each of these explanations is examined for understanding the sharp rise in drug prices.

Increases in Production Cost

An increase in production cost requires a producer to increase prices if it is to survive. The costs related to discovering and bringing to market a

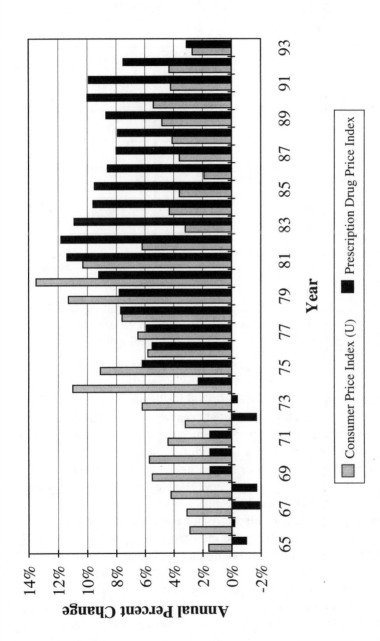

Note: CPI (U) = consumer price index for all urban consumers.
Sources: U.S. Bureau of the Census (Washington, DC), *Statistical Abstract of the United States* and *Historical Abstract of the United States,* various editions.

Figure 20.2   Direct Patient Payments as a Percentage of Health Care
Expenditures by Selected Categories, 1991

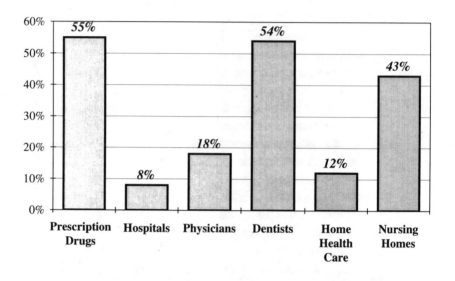

Sources: Health Care Financing Administration, Office of the Actuary/Office of National Health Statistics and the Agency for Health Care Policy and Research, *National Medical Expenditure Survey.*

new drug have risen greatly. The 1962 amendments to the Food, Drug, and Cosmetic Act (which were enacted because of the thalidomide scare) imposed more stringent testing requirements on drug companies before they are permitted to market a new drug. It now takes an average of 12 years from initial research to final drug approval. In 1987 it cost an estimated $231 million to bring a new drug to market; by 1995 these costs are expected to be $400 million.

Economies of scale in research and development (R and D) and in marketing costs are changing the industry's structure by reducing the number of drug firms that are competing with one another. In the R and D phase, many drug discoveries are eliminated before even one is determined to be safe and therapeutically better than other drugs. Drug companies are merging since they need large research budgets to tide them over through all the "dry holes" that must be explored before they can produce and bring to market a profitable drug. Only two out of every ten drugs developed receive FDA approval, and of these, only three of every ten recover their R and D costs. A small company is usually unable to sustain itself until it can finally reap the profits of a breakthrough drug. The potential for high earnings are needed if companies are going to invest large sums in R and D.

High R and D costs, however, are not the reason for high or rising drug prices. Large fixed or "sunk" costs are costs that have already been incurred; hence they are not relevant for setting a drug's price. It is true that fixed costs must eventually be recovered; otherwise, the drug company will lose money. However, the most profitable price to charge is based on the purchaser's willingness to pay and the drug's variable or "marginal" costs, that is, the actual costs of producing that drug. Unless the price is at least as high as the drug's variable costs, the drug company will not produce the drug. Variable costs typically include the manufacturing and distribution costs of a particular drug. Variable costs of branded drugs, however, are only a small fraction of their selling price, as evidenced by the low price at which generic drugs are sold. Rising drug prices, therefore, are not the result of sharply increasing variable costs.

Changing Demand Conditions

When costs do not explain price levels, then it becomes necessary to look at the demand for drugs, namely, how much people are willing to pay for a particular drug. If patients become less price sensitive because they now have prescription drug insurance, producers could increase their prices and reap greater profits; any loss in sales would be more than offset by the higher prices. Between the late 1960s to today, prescription drug insurance increased from 12 percent to 45 percent of total purchases. Increased outpatient drug coverage undoubtedly led to higher retail drug prices. Many patients and their physicians became less concerned with price differences and more likely to use well-advertised brand names when equally effective but less-expensive generic drugs are available.

There are, however, two markets for prescription drugs: the retail market (which serves individual patients) and large purchasers (such as HMOs, mail-order drug firms, and hospital purchasing groups). A growing number of patients with drug insurance belong to managed care organizations (HMOs and PPOs) whose physicians have incentives to be price sensitive and knowledgeable about the drugs they prescribe. The prices drug companies charge purchasers in these two markets differ, primarily because the groups differ in their willingness to pay; drug prices in the retail market will exceed those paid by large purchasers.

(For a recent review article on many of the issues covered in this chapter, see Scherer 1993.)

Of growing importance to the market for prescription drugs are the large purchasers. These organizations are establishing drug formularies—a list of prescription drugs from which their physicians must prescribe. As HMOs and PPOs seek volume discounts from drug companies, they are willing to limit their subscribers' choice of drugs in return for negotiating lower drug prices. Drug formulary committees focus on drugs where there are therapeutic substitutes and evaluate different drugs according to their therapeutic value and their price; higher-priced drugs are used only when justified by greater therapeutic benefits. Restrictions are then placed on their physicians' prescribing behavior. These organizations are also using computer technology to conduct drug utilization review; each physician's prescription is instantly checked against the formulary, and data are gathered on the performance of each physician as well as on the health plan's use of specific drugs.

Contracts between large purchasers and drug companies are expected to account for two-thirds of U.S. prescription drug sales by 1995. The availability of "me too" drugs contributes to price competition, as large purchasers have more choice and are able to switch brands to receive greater price concessions.

Improved Drugs

As managed care organizations evaluate drugs for inclusion in their formulary based on therapeutic benefits and price, differences in drug prices will reflect differences in therapeutic benefits. Knowledgeable purchasers, evaluating a higher-priced new drug, would only be willing to pay a higher price if the new drug's therapeutic benefits were greater than the older drug. New, higher-priced drugs will fail commercially if their therapeutic benefits are similar to existing drugs.

A new drug, for which there is no close substitute, and that is clearly therapeutically superior to existing drugs, will be higher priced. Approving an existing drug for a new use also increases its value, since its therapeutic effects for that new use are greater than existing drugs; the drug company is thus able to increase its price. The price of a new drug is determined by a purchaser's willingness to pay for its greater therapeutic benefits, rather than the cost of producing the drug.[1] Rising drug prices are, therefore, also an indication that new drugs are more effective than existing drugs.

As new, therapeutically improved drugs come on the market, the Bureau of Labor Statistics (BLS) drug price index should adjust the price of prescription drugs *downward* to account for improvements in their therapeutic benefits. Price indexes are supposed to measure inflation in the *same* goods and services sold in two different time periods. Unfortunately, the BLS treats the higher prices of new drugs as pure price increases (Cleeton, Goepfrich, and Weisbrod 1992). Had the BLS adjusted the price of prescription drugs down because of quality improvements (and generic substitutes when they become available) the drug price index shown in Figure 20.1 would not have risen as sharply during the 1980s. Consequently, drug price increases were greatly overstated during the 1980s.[2]

Based on the above discussion, the likely reasons for rising drug prices during the 1980s were increased outpatient drug coverage, which made patients less price sensitive, and the failure of the BLS drug price index to adjust for therapeutically improved drugs (and new generic substitutes). Cost increases are unlikely to have been an important contributor to rapidly rising drug prices.

Enacted and Proposed Legislation on Prescription Drugs

Regardless of whether a more accurate drug price index would have shown smaller price increases, the drug industry would still have come under political scrutiny. States are having difficulty in financing their rapidly increasing Medicaid expenditures, and rising drug expenditures are adding to these difficulties. Further, Medicare does not cover outpatient prescription drugs, the elderly take multiple prescriptions, and drugs for certain chronic conditions are very expensive. The aged also live on fixed incomes and account for a third of all retail prescription drugs; even though drugs are only 8 percent of total medical expenditures, they are a large percent of a patient's total out-of-pocket payments.

Several types of legislation have been enacted, and others proposed, to deal with these concerns of high out-of-pocket drug expenses and increasing Medicaid drug costs.

Limitation of Prescription Drugs
Available to Medicaid Patients

To lower their Medicaid expenditures, several states have limited Medicaid patients' prescription drug choices. Unfortunately, in some cases these restrictions are more concerned with the elimination of expensive drugs rather than the relative therapeutic benefits of different drugs. Elimination of expensive new drugs from state Medicaid drug formularies can result in higher medical expenditures per Medicaid recipient by causing an increase in hospital admissions and physician visits.

Expensive drugs can achieve large savings by reducing the length of a hospital stay or by eliminating the necessity for very costly surgical procedures. New antiulcer drugs, for example, cost about $1,000 a year, but they save $25,000 by reducing the need for surgery. Similarly, anti–heart attack drugs may cost $1,000, but they are much less costly than $30,000 for open-heart surgery.

Medicaid programs should have the same goal as managed care organizations, namely, reducing a patient's total medical expenditures rather than just reducing drug expenditures. Medicaid formularies should evaluate not only the price of a drug but its therapeutic benefits and its effect on the use of other medical services.

Prescription Drug Purchases for Medicaid at Volume Purchasers' Prices

At a federal level, Senator David Pryor (D-Ark.) sponsored legislation, enacted in 1990, that requires drug companies to sell drugs to Medicaid programs at their "best" prices offered to large volume purchasers. Until 1990, drugs prescribed for Medicaid patients were purchased by the patients at local pharmacies, and the Medicaid program was charged retail prices for the prescriptions. Because these prescriptions were purchased in thousands of local pharmacies by individual patients, Medicaid, which accounts for as much as 15 percent of drug sales, did not receive volume discounts as did the Veterans Administration, HMOs, or other large bulk drug purchasers. Forcing drug companies to give volume discounts to non-volume purchasers has had the predictable effect of drug companies raising their prices to volume purchasers.

Drug prices are lower to large purchasers because (1) it is less costly for drug companies to sell drugs in bulk to large purchasers and (2) large purchasers are willing to establish therapeutic review committees to evaluate different drugs and limit their patients' drug choices, which enables them to negotiate larger purchases based on the best price. For Medicaid programs to receive the same price savings, they must be able to engage in similar bulk purchasing.

Price Controls

The Clinton administration has discussed placing price controls on new breakthrough drugs both as a means of limiting patients' high out-of-pocket drug expenses and also for lowering the financing costs of including a prescription drug benefit in Medicare.

As evidence of the benefits of price controls, its proponents claim that drug prices in the United States are as much as 32 percent higher than the same drugs sold in Canada. Other countries use price controls and their purchasing power (threats of delisting a drug) to get price reductions from U.S. drug companies (U.S. General Accounting Office 1992).

Simple comparisons of drug prices between countries, however, cannot be easily made. Merely comparing the prices of drugs sold in retail pharmacies is a misleading indication of average drug prices. Drug companies in the United States sell to large bulk purchasers, such as HMOs, hospital purchasing groups, mail-order firms, the government, as well as to retail pharmacies. Price comparisons must also be adjusted for package size, strength of each dosage, and mix of dosage forms (tablets, liquid, delayed release); otherwise, the results are not comparable. Many countries also permit earlier adoption of new drugs that are substitutes to existing drugs, thereby creating greater price competition; in the United States it takes longer to introduce a new drug because FDA approval takes longer.

Some countries, particularly less-developed countries, either do not recognize United States patent protection laws or award patents for shorter periods than the United States. In countries where price controls on drugs exist, drug companies may still find it profitable to sell their drugs there since any profit can be used to offset the R and D expenses incurred in the United States. The small percent of total drug sales by these countries enables them to "free ride" on the R and D investments made by the drug firms in the United States.

However, if the United States were to implement price controls, either because of faulty comparisons between countries or because smaller countries are able to "free ride," there would be a large effect on the development of new drugs. Total drug expenditures would also increase, not decrease.

Drug price controls will lower drug firms' profitability, which in turn will reduce the rate of return from R and D investments, and consequently result in lower R and D expenditures. Biotechnology firms will have less incentive to invest in new miracle drugs since they will have less of a chance of making large profits. With fewer new drugs being developed, the public will be worse off; the quality of life for many will go down. And with fewer new drugs coming on the market, existing drugs will face less price competition and will be able to maintain higher prices for a longer period. Total health expenditures will be higher than if drug companies invested more in R and D and developed new drugs that reduced the costs of medical treatments. One of the most internationally competitive industries in the United States would be weakened.

The following example illustrates why price controls are not a solution to rising medical costs. Drugs are 8 percent, or about $72 billion, of total medical expenditures, which in 1992 were approximately $900 billion. Even reducing the annual rate of increase in drug prices (7 percent in 1992) to zero by imposing price controls would only save $5 billion a year ($72 billion multiplied by 7 percent). This savings is very small in relation to the annual increase in medical expenditures, which is approximately 10 percent, or $90 billion a year. More importantly, drug price controls would reduce drug firms' R and D, which are 16 percent of sales (roughly $11 billion).

Drug price controls offer limited potential for saving money and carry the risk of reducing R and D, 42 percent of which is for basic research; the remainder is spent on "me too" drugs. Why then do some legislators favor price controls? Politicians try to provide their constituents with short-term visible benefits at seemingly no cost. Since the controlled price would be higher than variable costs, drug firms would continue to sell their current drugs. The only apparent loser under drug price controls would be the drug companies. However, over time drug firms would undertake less R and D, but these longer-term effects of reduced mortality and improved quality of life are not obvious to the public nor will they be felt for some time.

There is some evidence of the effects that drug price controls have had on other countries. First, and most important, other countries' regulation of drug prices resulted in a decline in research and development of new drugs by drug firms in those countries. Second, drug expenditures increased and represent a higher portion of total medical expenditures in these countries (see Figure 20.3). In Germany, for example, low drug prices have increased patients' use of drugs so much that drugs represent 22 percent of total health expenditures. To reduce drug expenditures, the German government recently imposed financial penalties on physicians to limit their prescribing of too many drugs.

Figure 20.3   Pharmaceuticals as a Percentage of Total Health Care Expenditures in Different Countries, 1990

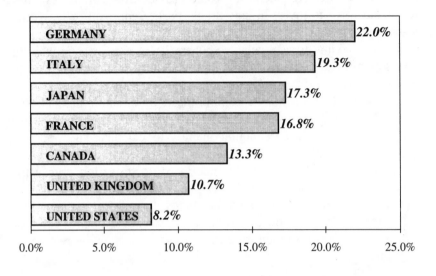

Source: Organization for Economic Cooperation and Development (OECD) (Paris, France).

Recommended Public Policies for Prescription Drugs

If regulation of drug prices and restrictive Medicaid formularies (eliminating new high-priced drugs) are unlikely to achieve either the short-term goal of minimizing total treatment expenditures or the longer-term goal of encouraging the development of therapeutically superior drugs, what public policies would be more appropriate?

Quicker FDA Approval of New Drugs

First, the FDA should provide quicker approval of new drugs. The availability of therapeutically superior new drugs could reduce treatment costs by substituting for more costly medical treatment and improve medical outcomes. Faster approval of new drugs will increase price competition with existing drugs. Quicker approval would also reduce the R and D costs of developing a new drug, since the drug company would receive a return on its investment sooner. Similarly, the profitability of a new drug would increase because there would be more years of patent life remaining after the drug is on the market. Lowering R and D costs and increasing the effective patent life would provide drug companies with a greater incentive to invest in new drugs. Earlier approval of new drugs by the FDA for AIDS patients occurred because of political pressure to make lifesaving drugs available sooner. There is no reason why this more streamlined process of drug approval should not be followed for all new drugs.

Drug safety need not be compromised by streamlining FDA approval. Drug companies should still be held liable for drug safety, which would make it in their economic interest to calculate the trade-offs between the potential loss from lawsuits from adverse drug effects and the revenues of a therapeutically superior drug. Ensuring drug safety would shift away from extensive, lengthy, and expensive pretesting to meet specified FDA testing requirements, followed by minimal FDA monitoring of drug use once it is released, toward a greater emphasis by drug companies on monitoring their drugs once they are released to the public.

Enrollment of Medicaid and Medicare Patients in Managed Care Organizations

The second change needed to improve the performance of the drug prescription market is for the government to encourage Medicaid and Medicare beneficiaries to enroll in managed care organizations. Large purchasers, such as third party insurers and managed care organizations, are placing greater emphasis on drug utilization mechanisms that develop profiles on physicians' prescribing patterns and on patients' use of drugs. Such drug utilization systems can serve to educate physicians regarding their prescribing patterns. Patient drug use profiles can serve to determine patient compliance with drug prescriptions, and they can enlighten physicians as to the medical outcomes associated with different drug therapies. These drug data systems could also serve as a monitoring mechanism for drug safety and enable evaluations to be made of the relative therapeutic benefits of different drugs.

Drug utilization data systems are more likely to be adopted by managed care organizations since they have an incentive to be concerned with medical outcomes and total medical expenditures per subscriber. Enrolling Medicaid and Medicare patients into managed care organizations would provide those patients with these same benefits and would eliminate the need for the government to reduce its Medicaid drug expenditures by regulating drug prices or by restricting access to new drugs.

Summary

The prescription drug market is changing, from one in which independent, fee-for-service physicians decide on the prescription and the patient purchases the drug at retail prices, to one in which drug companies market directly to managed care organizations. It is becoming less profitable for drug companies to rely on detail people to educate individual physicians about their drugs. Large drug purchasers are relying on their therapeutic review committees to evaluate the trade-off between the relative therapeutic benefits and higher prices of new drugs. A managed care environment wherein competition is based on annual premiums, medical outcomes, and patient satisfaction will have beneficial effects on the market for prescription drugs.

As the market for prescription drugs becomes more price competitive, rising drug prices should be welcomed, since they will be an indication that the therapeutic benefits of new drugs exceed those of lower-priced, older drugs. The public's concern should not be with whether drug company profits are high or drug prices are rising rapidly, but whether medical outcomes are improved by the use of new drugs and whether total medical treatment costs are reduced.

Notes

1. According to the 1962 drug amendments, a new drug must not only be safe (according to FDA testing requirements) but must also be "effective," meaning the drug must achieve the manufacturer's claims. Thus, since 1962, for a new drug to be approved by the FDA, the manufacturer must offer proof that it is therapeutically better than existing drugs.
2. The BLS drug price index further overstates drug price increases when a generic equivalent of a branded drug comes on the market. The lower-priced generic drug rapidly expands its market share at the expense of the branded drug, for which it is a substitute. The price of the branded drug often increases as it loses market share because the remaining patients are less price sensitive and they believe the branded drug is higher in quality and are therefore reluctant to use the generic version of the drug. The BLS picks up the price increase of the branded drug, but it does not measure the price decline experienced by the large proportion of consumers who switch

to the generic version. Thus the BLS drug price index fails to reflect the sharp price decline with the introduction of the generic drug.

References

Cleeton, D., V. Goepfrich, and B. Weisbrod. "What Does the Consumer Price Index for Prescription Drugs Really Measure?" *Health Care Financing Review*. 13 (Spring 1992): 45–51.

Scherer, F. M. "Pricing, Profits, and Technological Progress in the Pharmaceutical Industry." *Journal of Economic Perspectives* 7 (Summer 1993): 97–115.

U.S. General Accounting Office. *Prescription Drug Charges in U.S. and Canada.* GAO/HRD-92-110. Washington, DC: U.S. General Accounting Office, 1992.

21

Should Kidneys (and Other Organs) Be Bought and Sold?

Between 1988 and 1992 more than 10,000 people died waiting for an organ transplant. During this same period, the number of people waiting for a transplant rose 66 percent, to 49,933, while the number of organs donated increased just 31 percent, to 15,000 (see Figure 21.1). More than 80 percent of those waiting for organ transplants are waiting for kidney transplants; the remainder are for heart, liver, lung, and pancreas organs. The number of people dying each year while waiting for an organ transplant is increasing.

Even though the total number of transplants is increasing each year (as shown in Figure 21.2), the gap between those waiting for organ transplants and the supply of organs has been growing rapidly as more patients are being recommended for such transplants. The discovery of immunosuppressive drugs to reduce the risk of rejection has greatly increased the success rate of organ transplants; success rates for kidney transplants have increased from approximately 60 percent to 96 percent. Unfortunately, there is an insufficient number of organs to keep up with the growing demand. The consequence is that many of those waiting for a transplant will die before an organ becomes available.

Patients waiting for a kidney transplant (the most common organ transplant) must rely on kidney dialysis, which is in itself costly. It has been estimated that if all those patients on dialysis and waiting for a transplant could be given a kidney transplant, the federal government, which pays for kidney dialysis and kidney transplants under Medicare,

217

Figure 21.1   Demand for Organs and the Total Number of Organs
Donated, 1988–1992

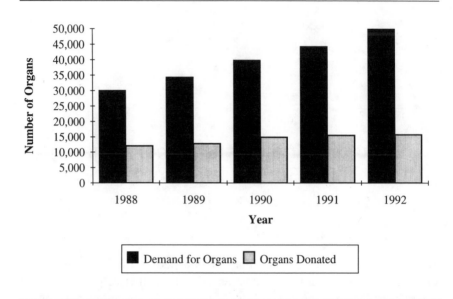

Source: U.S. General Accounting Office Report to Congressional Committees, *Organ Transplants; Increased Effort Needed to Boost Supply and Ensure Equitable Distribution of Organs* (Washington, DC), April 1993, 68.

could save approximately $1 billion over a five-year period. Kidney transplantation is a lower-cost form of treatment than dialysis. In addition to being higher cost, dialysis takes time, up to seven hours per day, for several days a week. Kidney dialysis patients have a reduced quality of life, as well as lower productivity.[1]

Sources of Organs for Transplant

There are two sources of supply for organ transplants: living donors, such as family members who donate one of their kidneys, and cadavers. Approximately 80 percent of kidney organs, as well as all other organs used for transplants, such as hearts, lungs, and livers, come from victims who have just been killed in an accident.

The motivating force upon which transplant patients have long depended is altruism. It is illegal (according to the National Organ Transplant Act of 1984) to purchase or sell human organs. Current efforts to

Figure 21.2   Number of Organ Transplants, Selected Years, 1981–1992

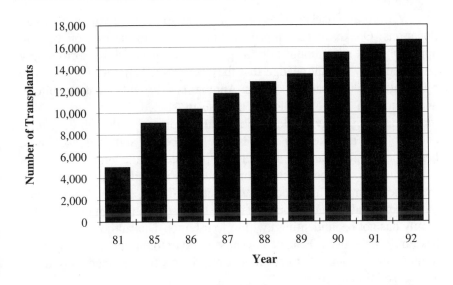

Note: Figures include heart, liver, kidney, heart-lung, lung, and pancreas transplants.
Sources: U.S. Bureau of the Census (Washington, DC), *Statistical Abstract of the United States, 1992,* and United Network for Organ Sharing, Research Department (Richmond, VA).

increase the supply of organs rely on approaches to stimulate voluntary organ donations by the deceased's family members.

Currently, the family of the deceased is asked by medical personnel, shortly after they have been notified of the death of a family member, to donate their loved one's body organs. Physicians are often reluctant to make such a request to a grieving family, and the grieving family is reluctant to agree while still shocked by the death of a loved one. For some families the sorrow might be somewhat offset by the belief that another person's life might be saved. However, only a small fraction of families are willing to give permission for their deceased family member's organs to be used for transplant patients. For reasons that are psychological, such as the thought of dismemberment of a loved one, and religious, families of the deceased are reluctant to donate the deceased's organs. The time period in which such a request can be made is short; otherwise, the organ will deteriorate. The family must be located, permission must be received, a recipient must be located through the national organ network, and a tissue match made between the recipient and the deceased.

Various approaches have been proposed to increase voluntary organ donations. One is to use improved "marketing" techniques on how to approach (and who should talk to) grieving families, whose sorrow may be lessened by the knowledge that they have saved another person's life by donating the deceased's organs. Another is to provide greater publicity and education to the public on the use of signed donor cards, which make their organs available to potential recipients. Although education and publicity are likely to increase the number of signed donor cards, hence potential organs, it is still the practice of the organ transplant community to seek permission from the donor's family before harvesting the donor's organ. In some states, such as Texas, medical authorities have been legally granted permission to harvest organs from bodies if the family has not been identified within four hours. This authority, however, has rarely been used. Fear of lawsuits, unfavorable publicity, and desire to maintain the public's trust prevent physicians from immediately using a deceased donor's organs.

"Presumed consent" laws have been proposed that would make the deceased's organs available unless the deceased or their family had previously opposed it. These laws, which are in force in many European countries, have not increased organ donation rates greater than in the United States, presumably for the same reasons permission is still sought for signed donor cards.

Waiting for permission from the deceased's family often results in the organs being lost. Although about 20,000 people who die each year have organs suitable for harvesting, such as those who die in accidents, only a small percent of those organs are actually donated. Under the current system of altruism, the supply of donors has increased very slowly, from 5,877 in 1988 to 6,800 in 1991.

Donor Compensation Proposals

The growing imbalance between supply and demand for organs has led some persons to advocate compensating donors to increase the supply of donated organs. Compensating donors (or their families) is highly controversial and would require a change in current legislation prohibiting the purchase or sale of body organs. Organ payment proposals cover the spectrum from the so-called mild—paying family members for organs of their deceased kin—to "strong"—paying a living donor for their second kidney. The following discussion covers three such proposals.

Compensating Families after Death of the Donor

It has been proposed that the burial costs of the deceased be paid if the family permits the harvesting of the deceased's organs. Similarly, the family of the deceased could be paid an amount varying between $1,000 and $5,000. A potential problem with these proposals is that it may be awkward at the time of death to negotiate a financial transaction with families traumatized by the death of a loved one. Another possible problem is that organ purchases of the deceased, which would presumably be directed toward those with low incomes, might offend low-income minority families, who might feel that they are being exploited to benefit wealthy White individuals.

Compensating Donors before Death

Allowing individuals to sell their organs in advance of their death has the advantage that family members would not be subject to the psychological and social pressure to make a quick decision at the time they are suffering the loss of a loved one. Thus a second approach is to allow individuals to sell the rights to their organs if they were to die in return for a reduction in their health or auto insurance premiums. Health or automobile insurance companies might offer their subscribers, annually, a choice of lower premiums to those who are willing to donate their organs if they were to die during the coming year. The insurance company would then have the right to harvest (sell) the deceased organs during the period of the insurance contract. Each of the potential donors would then be listed in a central computer registry, which a hospital would check when a patient died. Transplant recipients would also be listed in a national registry, and their health insurer or the government would reimburse the insurer a previously stated price for the organ.

For example, if the value of all of a deceased's organs were worth $100,000 at time of death, and the probability of dying during the year was 10,000 to 1 (the current average chance of dying during a year), then the annual premium reduction would be $10. If the value of all the organs were greater than $100,000 or the probability of death lower than 10,000 to 1, the premium reduction would be greater. Young drivers and motorcyclists would presumably be offered large automobile insurance reductions.

The price of organs could either be established competitively or by the government establishing a price, for example, $10,000 for a kidney. These prices would then be used by the insurance company, together with the probability that the subscriber will die during the next year, to establish the annual premium reduction for the potential donor. If too few insurance subscribers were willing to accept the premium reduction, then the price of the organ (if established by the government) could be increased until the likely supply is large enough to satisfy the estimated demand for transplants. The greater the shortage of organs, the larger will be the reductions in insurance premiums for organ donors.

Paying Living Kidney Donors

The most controversial approach for increasing the supply of organs is to pay living donors a sufficiently high price for them to part with one of their kidneys. Paying a market price to bring forth an increase in supply is already occurring in other highly sensitive areas of human behavior, such as with the use of sperm banks and surrogate mothers, who are willing to be impregnated with another couple's fertilized egg in return for a fee.

Market transactions consist of a voluntary exchange of assets between two parties. People engage in voluntary exchange because they differ in their valuation of the asset and they both expect to benefit from the transaction. If sales of kidneys were permitted, the person selling the kidney would receive a fee that he or she believes would compensate them for the loss of their kidney. The purchaser believes that the kidney is worth at least what they are willing to pay for it. The purchaser is unlikely to be an individual; it is likely to be the government, since kidney transplants are covered under Medicare, in which case paying for the kidney would be similar to paying the surgeon for the operation. No one is made worse off by voluntary trade. Thus the first major advantage of legalizing the sale of kidneys is that no one is worse off and it is likely that both are better off with the voluntary exchange than when it is prohibited.

There are other important advantages to permitting a commercial market for kidneys. Organs can be purchased that would save the lives of all those waiting for a kidney. No longer would they have to endure the suffering that occurs while waiting for a kidney donation and possibly die before one becomes available. Further, the government would save a great deal of money by substituting kidney transplants for kidney dialysis, since a transplant is a lower-cost method of treatment than dialysis, which is the current form of treatment for those waiting for transplants. Lastly, there would be an increase in the quality of donated kidneys, which would increase the success rate of the transplant. Currently, donated kidneys are used that do not have good tissue matches because of the severe shortage of kidneys. Paying living donors for their kidneys would result in more choice of donors, thereby enabling tissue matches between recipient and donor to be made in advance.

Opposition to Financial Incentives to Organ Donation

Opposition to using financial incentives for increasing the supply of organs is based on several reasons. First, there is the belief that using financial incentives would discourage voluntary donations of organs, thereby resulting in a smaller supply of organs. The only evidence that may be indicative of what is likely to happen to the overall supply of organs when financial incentives are offered is to examine what happened when financial incentives were used for increasing the supply of blood. Voluntary donations of blood declined, but the decline was more than offset by an increase in the supply of paid donations.

Second, it is claimed that paying living donors for their organs would exploit the poor to benefit the wealthy; the poor are likely to be the sellers of organs, while those with higher incomes would be the beneficiaries. The poor, it is claimed, would be forced to sell their organs to provide for their families. However, if the poor have inadequate funds, then this is because society is unwilling to provide them with sufficient subsidies to either increase their incomes or to provide them with education that would increase their productivity and incomes. Prohibiting the poor from selling one of their assets will leave them worse off; they are prevented from doing something that they believe will improve their situation.

Although little risk is involved in selling one's kidney, a donor will be accepting a slightly higher risk of dying in return for increased financial rewards. Many people seek additional compensation by choosing to work in higher-risk occupations. There are occupational risks when working in a coal mine, on a skyscraper, or on an off-shore drilling platform, and yet society does not interfere with these voluntary transactions.

Someone willing to make the trade-off between greater compensation and the loss of a kidney is not "forced" to sell their organs.

There is the concern that those selling their kidney might be subject to fraud and that they will then regret selling their kidney. Various protections could be included in legislation legalizing the sale of kidneys. A waiting period, such as six months, could be used in case the person decides to change his or her mind. The donor could also be required to be of a minimum age. Also, the donor must be approved by a panel that includes a psychiatrist or social worker to assess the donor's ability to make rational choices.

Whenever demand exceeds supply in a market, prices rise. When prices are not permitted to rise or are illegal, then there is the potential for a black market. Although the sale of kidney organs in the United States is illegal, a wealthy patient has access to an international black market, particularly from donors from less-developed countries, such as India and China. Demand for kidney organs is lower when the activity is illegal than if sales were legal. There are higher search costs to find an organ donor on the black market, purchasers are less certain of the organ's quality, there are no legal remedies if fraud occurs, and the purchaser would have to pay the hospital's and surgeon's costs out-of-pocket. However, it is an option available to the wealthy. Prohibiting the sale of organs thus again discriminates against the poor, who do not have access to the international black market in kidney organs.

If a legal market in organs were permitted, would only the wealthy be able to afford kidney transplants once the price of a kidney is included in the already high price of a transplant? The answer is no. Kidney transplants are currently paid for by the federal government; thus the higher cost would not be a deterrent to any recipient needing a transplant. Most of the costs for a transplant are for hospital and physician services; including the price of the organ would not be a large addition to those costs. Currently, everyone associated with the transplant benefits—the recipient receives a new kidney and the physician and hospital receive payment for their services. Why shouldn't the donor also benefit?

What if a low-income person, desperate for money, sells his or her kidney and subsequently suffers from kidney disease? Since the government currently pays for all kidney transplants as part of Medicare, that donor would then become eligible for a free transplant. A new donor would be paid for a kidney to be used for the previous donor's transplant.

Would the opponents of a compensation system who are concerned with its effects on the poor be more positively inclined to using financial incentives if the poor (defined, for example, as those with incomes below the federal poverty level) were prohibited from selling their organs? Would the poor be better off if they were denied the right to sell one of their assets? It is paternalistic to believe that society helps the poor when those with higher incomes limit their choices.

The poor and minority groups are currently disadvantaged by the present "altruistic" system for securing and allocating organs. Many of those waiting for transplants have low incomes. Further, although Blacks are (statistically) more likely to suffer from kidney disease than Whites, they are less likely to receive an organ transplant. Blacks comprise one-third of the waiting list for kidney transplants. The reason for the higher proportion of Blacks on the waiting list is that Black kidney patients have a low tissue match with Whites and Blacks donate proportionately fewer kidneys than Whites (*Wall Street Journal* 1993).

The growing demand for transplants, together with its profitability to both the hospital and the surgeon, has resulted in more hospitals becoming "transplant" centers. According to a Government Accounting Office report, the competition among these transplant centers for organs has resulted in a situation whereby organs are not transferred nationally or regionally to those hospitals who have had patients waiting the longest or who are most in need. The result has been a less-efficient allocation system and an increase in deaths among those patients at hospitals that are less able to increase the number of voluntary donations. As the feasibility of transplants increases and as more hospitals and physicians find status and profit in performing transplants, the shortage of voluntary organs and its consequences will become more severe.

Perhaps the strongest objection to compensating donors for their organs are some people's ideological and moral beliefs. Financial incentives, governed by greed, would substitute for altruism as the motivating force for donating one's organs. This is deeply offensive to many persons. No decision, however, is without costs. There is a trade-off that must be considered. While the thought of having people sell their organs is offensive, thousands of people will die each year for lack of a kidney donor, and this number will increase. Which choice is more offensive—violating the strongly held beliefs of some persons regarding the repugnance of a market for human organs versus the suffering and loss of lives of thousands of people needing an organ transplant?

Note

1. The discussion in this chapter is based on Hansmann 1989. See also U.S. General Accounting Office 1993.

References

Hansmann, H. "The Economics and Ethics of Markets for Human Organs." *Journal of Health Politics, Policy and Law* 14 (Spring 1989): 57–85.

U.S. General Accounting Office. *Organ Transplants: Increased Effort Needed to Boost Supply to Ensure Equitable Distribution of Organs.* GAO/HRD-93-56. Washington, DC: U.S. General Accounting Office, 1993.

Wall Street Journal. "Tissue Typing in Kidney Transplants Is Said to Hurt Black Patients' Chances." (1 April 1993): A6.

22

The Role of Government in Medical Care

Government intervention in the financing and delivery of medical services is pervasive. On the financing side, hospital and physician services for the aged are subsidized (Medicare); there is a separate Social Security tax to pay for those subsidies; Medicaid is a federal/state matching program to pay for medical services for the poor; there is a large network of state and county hospitals; health professional education schools are subsidized; there are government-guaranteed loan programs for students in the health professions; employer-paid health insurance is excluded from taxable income; there is a separate medical program for veterans; the Civilian Health and Medical Program of the Uniformed Services (CHAMPUS) finances health benefits for military dependents; and medical research is subsidized. These are some of the programs that make government a 40 percent partner in total health expenditures.

In addition to these financing programs, extensive government regulations influence the financing and delivery of medical services. For example, state licensing boards determine the criteria for entry into the different professions, practice acts determine which tasks can be performed by various professional groups, in some states hospital payment is regulated while in other states hospital investment is subject to state review, hospital and physician prices under Medicare are regulated, health insurance companies are regulated by the states, each state sets mandates as to what benefits (e.g., hair transplants in Minnesota) and which providers (e.g., naturopaths in California) should be included in health insurance sold in their state, and some states have required employers to provide health insurance benefits to their employees.

The role of government in the financing and delivery of medical services, as well as through federal and state regulation, is extensive. To understand the reasons for these different types of government intervention and, at times, seemingly contradictory policies, it becomes necessary to have a view of what the government is attempting to achieve.

The Public Interest View of Government

The traditional or public interest role of government can be classified according to its policy objectives and the policy instruments to achieve those objectives. The policy objectives of government in the health field are twofold: (1) to redistribute medical resources to those least able to purchase medical services and (2) to improve the economic efficiency by which medical services are purchased and delivered. These traditional objectives of government, redistribution and efficiency, can be achieved by using one or more of the following policy instruments: expenditures, taxation, and regulation. The policy instruments can be applied to either the purchaser (demand) or the supplier side of the market. These policy objectives and instruments, which can be used to classify each type of government health policy according to policy objectives, the type of policy instrument used, and whether the policy instrument is directed toward the demand or supply side of the market, are shown in Table 22.1.

Redistribution

Redistribution causes a change in wealth. According to the public interest view of government, society makes a value judgment that medical services should be provided to those with low incomes and financed by taxing those with higher incomes. Redistributive programs typically lower the cost of services to a particular group by enabling them to purchase those services at below-market prices. These benefits are then financed by imposing a "cost" on some other group. Two large redistributive programs are Medicare for the aged and Medicaid for the medically indigent. The benefits and costs of a redistributive medical program, such as Medicaid, are shown in Table 22.2.

Table 22.1   Health Policy Objectives and Interventions

		Government Objectives	
Government Policy Instruments		*Redistribution*	*Improve Efficiency*
Expenditures	{ Demand side Supply side		
Taxation(+/−)	{ Demand side Supply side		
Regulation	{ Demand side Supply side		

Table 22.2   Determining the Redistributive Effects of Government Programs

	Low Income	*High Income*
Benefits	X	
Costs		X

Efficiency

The second traditional objective of government is to improve the efficiency with which society allocates resources. Inefficiency in resource allocation can occur, for example, when firms in a market have monopoly power or when externalities exist. A firm has monopoly power when it is able to charge a price that exceeds its cost by more than a normal profit. Monopoly is inefficient because it produces too small a level of service (output). The additional benefit to purchasers (as indicated by its price) from consuming a service is greater than the cost of producing that benefit; therefore more resources should flow into that industry until the additional benefit of consuming that service equals the additional cost of producing it.

The bases of monopoly power are several: there may be only one firm in a market, such as when there is a natural monopoly, for example, an electric company; there may be barriers to entry in a market; firms may collude on raising their prices; or because of a lack of information, consumers are unable to judge price, quality, and service differences among different suppliers. In each of these situations, the prices charged will exceed the costs of producing the product (which includes a normal profit). The appropriate government remedy to decrease monopoly power is to eliminate barriers to entry into a market, to prevent price collusion, and to improve information among consumers.

The second situation where the allocation of resources can be improved is when there are "externalities," which occur when someone undertakes an action and in so doing affects others who are not part of that transaction. The effects on others could be positive or negative. For example, a utility using high-sulfur coal to produce electricity also produces air pollution. As a result of the air pollution, residents in surrounding communities may have a higher incidence of respiratory illness. Resources are misallocated since the cost of producing electricity excludes the costs imposed on others. As a result, too much electricity is being produced. If the costs of producing electricity also included the costs imposed on others, the electricity price would be higher, and consequently its demand would be less. The allocation of resources would be improved if the utility's cost included both types of costs.

The appropriate role of government in such a situation is to determine the costs imposed on others and to tax the utility an equivalent amount. (This subject is discussed more completely in the following chapter.)

The Economic Theory of Regulation

Dissatisfaction with the public interest theory occurred for several reasons. Instead of just regulating natural monopolies, government has also regulated competitive industries, such as airlines, trucks, taxicabs, as well as various professions. Further, nonregulated firms always want to enter regulated markets. To prevent entry into regulated industries, the government establishes entry barriers. If the government supposedly reduces prices in regulated markets, and hence the firm's profitability, why should firms seek to enter a regulated industry?

To reconcile these apparent contradictions with the public interest view of government, an alternative theory of government behavior, the economic theory of regulation, was developed (Stigler 1971; for a more complete discussion of this theory and its applicability to the health field, see Feldstein 1988). The basic assumption underlying the economic theory is that political markets are no different from economic markets; individuals and firms seek to further their self-interest. Firms undertake investments in private markets to achieve a high rate of return. Why wouldn't the same firms invest in legislation if it also offered a high rate of return? Organized groups are willing to pay a price for legislative benefits. This price is political support, which brings together the demanders and suppliers of legislative benefits.

The Suppliers: Legislators

The suppliers of legislative benefits are legislators, and their goal is assumed to be to maximize their chances for reelection. As the late Senator Everett Dirksen said, "The first law of politics is to get elected, the second law is to be reelected." To be reelected requires political support, which consists of campaign contributions, votes, and volunteer time. Legislators are assumed to be rational, to make cost-benefit calculations when faced with demands for legislation. However, the legislator's cost-benefit calculations are not the costs and benefits to society of enacting particular legislation. Instead, the benefits are the additional political support the legislator would receive from supporting the legislation, and the costs are the lost political support they would incur as a result of their action. When the benefits to the legislators exceed their costs, they will support the legislation.

The Demanders: Those with a Concentrated Interest

Those who have a "concentrated" interest—that is, the legislation will have a large effect on their profitability, by either affecting their revenues or their costs—are more likely to be successful in the legislative marketplace. It becomes worthwhile for the group to organize, to represent their interests before legislators, and to raise political support to achieve the profits that favorable legislation can provide. It is for this reason that only those with a concentrated interest will demand legislative benefits.

Diffuse Costs

Whenever legislative benefits are provided to one group, others must bear those costs. When only one group has a concentrated interest in the legislation, they are more likely to be successful if the costs to finance those benefits are not obvious and can be spread over a large number of people. When this occurs, then the costs are said to be "diffuse." For example, assume that there are ten firms in an industry and, if they can have legislation enacted that would limit imports that compete with their products, they would be able to raise their prices and thereby receive $280 million in legislative benefits. These firms have a concentrated interest ($280 million) in trying to enact such legislation. The costs of these legislative benefits are financed by a small increase in the price of their product amounting to $1 per person. It is often not obvious to consumers that the legislation increases their costs. Further, even if consumers were aware of the legislation's effect, it would not be worthwhile for them to organize and represent their interests so as to forestall a price increase that will decrease their income by $1 a year. The costs of trying to prevent the cost increase would exceed their potential savings.

It is easier (less costly) for providers rather than consumers to organize, provide political support, and impose a diffuse cost on others. It is for this reason that there has been so much legislation affecting entry into the health professions, which tasks are reserved to certain professions, how (and which) providers are paid under public medical programs, why subsidies for medical education are given to the school and not to the student (otherwise they would have to compete for students), and so on. Most health issues have been relatively technical, such as the training of health professions, certification of their quality, methods of payment, controls on hospital capital investment, and so on. The higher medical prices resulting from regulations that benefit providers have been diffuse and not visible to consumers.

Entry Barriers to Regulated Markets

The economic theory of legislation provides an explanation for the above dissatisfactions with the public interest theory. Firms in competitive markets seek regulation so as to earn higher profits than are available in competitive markets. Prices in regulated markets, such as interstate airline travel, were always higher than nonregulated markets, such as intrastate air travel, thereby enabling regulated firms to earn greater profits. These higher prices provided nonregulated firms with an incentive to try to enter regulated markets. Government, on behalf of the regulated industry, imposed entry barriers to keep out low-priced competitors. Otherwise, the regulated firms could not earn more than a competitive rate of return.

Firms try to receive through legislation the monopoly profits they were unable to achieve through market competition.

Opposing Concentrated Interests

When only one group has a concentrated interest in the outcome of legislation and the costs are diffuse, legislators will respond to the political support the group is willing to pay to have favorable legislation enacted. When there are opposing groups, each with a concentrated interest in the outcome, legislators are likely to reach a compromise between the competing demanders of legislative benefits. Rather than balancing the gain in political support from one group against the loss from the other, legislators prefer to receive political support from both groups and impose diffuse costs on those with little political support.

Visible Redistributive Effects

When the beneficiaries are specific population groups, such as the aged, the redistributive effects of the legislation are meant to be very visible. An example of this is Medicare. By making it clear which population groups will benefit, legislators hope to receive their political support. The costs of financing such visible redistributive programs, however, are still designed to be diffuse so as not to generate political opposition from others. A small diffuse tax imposed on many people, such as a sales and payroll tax, is the only way large sums of money can be raised, with little opposition, to finance visible redistributive programs. These taxes are regressive—the tax represents a greater portion of income from low-income employees and consumers. Economists have determined that payroll taxes, even when imposed on the employer, are borne mostly by the employee; by imposing part of the tax on the employer, however, it appears that employees are paying a smaller portion of it than they really are. The remainder of the tax is shifted forward to consumers in the form of higher prices for the goods and services they purchase.

Medicaid and Medicare

Differences in the sources of political support are important for understanding our two main redistributive programs. Medicaid is a means-tested program for the poor and is funded from general tax revenues.

Since the poor (who have low voting participation rates) are unable to provide legislators with political support, the support for Medicaid comes from the middle class, who must agree to higher taxes to provide the poor with medical benefits. The inadequacy of Medicaid in every state, the conditions necessary for achieving Medicaid eligibility, the low levels of eligibility, and their lack of access to medical providers are related to the generosity (or lack thereof) of the middle class. The beneficiaries of Medicare, on the other hand, are the aged themselves, who (together with their children) provide the political support for the program. As the cost of Medicare has risen, government has raised Social Security taxes and reduced payments to providers rather than reducing benefits or beneficiaries from this politically powerful group.

The political necessity of keeping costs diffuse explains why the financing of both Medicare and producer regulation uses regressive taxes, either payroll taxes or higher prices for medical services. Spreading the costs over large populations keeps those costs diffuse. The net effect is that low-income persons pay the costs and higher-income persons, such as physicians or high-income aged, receive the benefits. Those receiving the benefits and those bearing the costs, according to the economic theory, are not based on income, as shown in Table 22.2, but instead according to which groups are able to offer political support (the beneficiaries) and which groups are unable to do so (they bear the costs). Regressive taxes are typically used to finance producer regulation as well as provide benefits to specific population groups.

Changes in Health Policies

Health policies change over time because groups who previously bore a diffuse cost develop a concentrated interest. Until the 1960s, medical societies were the main group with a concentrated interest in the financing and delivery of medical services. Thus the delivery system was structured to benefit physicians. The physician-to-population ratio remained constant for 15 years (until the mid-1960s) at 141 per 100,000, state restrictions were imposed on HMOs to limit their development, advertising was prohibited, and restrictions were placed on other health professionals to limit their ability to compete with physicians. Financing mechanisms also benefited physicians; until the 1980s, capitation payment for HMOs was prohibited under Medicare and Medicaid, and competitors to physicians were excluded from reimbursement under public and private insurance systems.

As the costs of medical care continued to increase rapidly to government and employers, their previously diffuse costs became concentrated. Under Medicare, the government was faced with the choice of raising taxes or reducing benefits to the aged, both of which would have cost the administration political support. Successive administrations developed a concentrated interest in lowering the rate of increase in medical expenditures. Similarly, large employers were concerned that rising medical costs were making them less competitive internationally. The pressures for cost containment increased as the "costs" of an inefficient delivery and payment system grew larger. Rising medical expenditures are no longer a diffuse cost to large purchasers of medical services.

Other professional organizations, such as pyschologists, chiropractors, and podiatrists saw the potentially greater revenues their members could receive if they were better able to compete with physicians. These groups developed a concentrated interest in securing payment for their members under public and private insurance systems and expanding their scope of practice. The rise in opposing concentrated interests weakened the political influence of organized medicine.

Summary

The public interest and economic theories of government provide opposing predictions of the redistributive and efficiency effects of government legislation, as shown in Table 22.3. To determine which of these contrasting theories is a more accurate description of government, it is necessary to match the actual outcomes of legislation to each theory's predictions. Do the benefits of redistributive programs go to those with low incomes and are they financed by taxes that impose a larger burden on those with higher incomes? Does the government try and improve the allocation of resources by reducing barriers to entry and, in markets where information is limited, monitoring quality of physicians' and other medical services and making this information available?

The economic theory of regulation provides greater understanding of why health policies are enacted and why they have changed over time than alternative theories. The economic theory predicts that government is not concerned with efficiency issues. Redistribution is the main objective of government, but it is to redistribute wealth to those who are able to offer political support from those who are unable to do so. Thus the reason medical licensing boards are inadequately staffed, have

Table 22.3   Health Policy Objectives under Different Theories of Government

Theories of Government	Objective of Government	
	Redistribution	*Improve Efficiency*
Public Interest Theory	Assist those with low incomes	Remove (and prevent) monopoly abuses and protect environment (externalities)
Economic Theory of Regulation	Provide benefits to those able to deliver political support and finance from those having little political support	Efficiency objective unimportant; more likely to protect industries so as to provide them with redistributive benefits

never required reexamination for relicensure, and have failed to monitor practicing physicians is that organized medicine has been opposed to any approaches for increasing quality that would adversely affect physicians' incomes. Regressive taxes are used to finance programs such as Medicare, not because legislators are unaware of their regressive nature, but because it is in the economic interest of those who have a concentrated interest.

The structure and financing of medical services is rational; the participants act according to their calculation of costs and benefits. Viewed in its entirety, however, health policy is uncoordinated and seemingly contradictory. Health policies are inequitable and inefficient; low-income persons end up subsidizing those with higher incomes. These results, however, are the consequences of a rational system. The outcomes were the result of policies intended by the legislators.

References

Feldstein, P. J. *The Politics of Health Legislation: An Economic Perspective.* Ann Arbor, MI: The Health Administration Press, 1988.
Stigler, G. J. "The Economic Theory of Regulation." *The Bell Journal of Economics* 2 (Spring 1971): 3–21.

23

Medical Research, Medical Education, Alcohol Consumption, and Pollution: Who Should Pay?

An important role of government is to improve the way markets allocate resources. When markets perform poorly, fewer goods and services are produced and incomes are lower than they would be otherwise. The usual policy prescription for improving the performance of markets is for the government to eliminate barriers to entry and increase information. Competitive markets, where there are no entry barriers and purchasers and producers are fully informed, are likely to produce the "correct" (or optimal) rate of output. The correct rate occurs if individuals benefiting from the service pay the full costs of producing that service. Resources are optimally allocated when the additional benefits from consuming the last unit equal the cost of producing that last unit. When still more units are consumed, the costs of those additional units exceed the benefits provided, and it would be better to use the resources to produce other goods and services whose benefits exceed their costs. As shown in Figure 23.1, when the costs are C_1 and benefits are B_1, the correct rate of output is Q_1. The benefit curve is declining because the more one has of a good, the lower the value of an additional unit.

Under certain circumstances, however, even a competitive market may not allocate resources correctly. The optimal rate of output in a market occurs when all the costs and benefits are included. Private decision makers consider only their own costs and benefits and exclude the costs or benefits imposed on others, if any. The effect may be that

Figure 23.1   The "Correct" Rate of Output

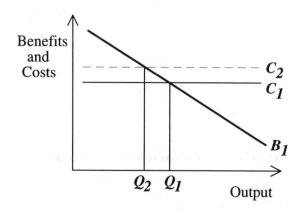

some services are "underproduced" while others are "overproduced." The reason the quantity of medical and health services may not be optimal is that costs and benefits may be imposed on persons other than those who purchase and provide the service. What happens, then, when costs or benefits are imposed on someone who is not a voluntary participant of that private transaction? Such "external" costs and benefits must be included; otherwise, either too much or too little of the service is produced and purchased. For example, when external costs are imposed on others, as shown by C_2 in Figure 23.1, then the correct rate of output declines from Q_1 to Q_2, which is where both private (C_1) and external costs (C_2) equal the benefits (B_1) from consuming that good or service.

When such external costs or benefits exist, government should calculate their magnitude, then use subsidies and taxes to achieve the "right" rate of output in the affected industry. Subsidies or taxes on the producers in that industry will change the costs of producing a service, so producers will adjust their level of output. The difference between C_1 and C_2, which is the external cost, is also the size of the tax to be imposed on each unit of the product.

Pollution

One reason externalities, such as pollution, occur is that no one owns the resource being exploited. Even if a resource, whether it be air or water, is scarce, if no one owns it, a firm may use it as though it were free; it does not become a cost of production as it would if the firm were charged a fee for its use. The lack of property rights over scarce resources is the basis for government intervention. For example, when a firm pollutes a stream in the process of producing its product, those who use that stream for recreational purposes are adversely affected; they bear a cost not included in the firm's calculation of its costs of producing the product. Since the firm has not had to include the external costs of production, it sells the product at a lower price, and the user pays less for that product than the product actually costs society. Because of its lower price, a greater quantity of the product is purchased and produced.

When there are no property rights over a scarce resource and it is used by large numbers of people and firms, negotiations among the parties over the use of that resource are likely to be difficult and costly. Government intervention is needed to calculate the external costs and, in the case of pollution, to impose a tax, equivalent to the amount of pollution caused, on each unit of the product sold. The product's higher price would include both the cost of production plus the unit tax; therefore less of the product would be sold. If all the costs and benefits, both private and external, were part of the private decision-making process, the industry would then produce the "right" rate of output.

A pollution tax could not be expected to eliminate all pollution, but it will reduce it to the correct level; the tax revenues received by the government would then go toward cleaning up the pollution or for compensating those who were adversely affected. If the government were to attempt to eliminate all the pollution, it would have to stop production of that product completely. Eliminating all pollution could adversely affect a great many people if the total benefits derived from that product outweigh its costs, including the costs of pollution. Consider, for example, the effect of eliminating all air pollution originating from automobiles or from producing electricity. Clearly, people prefer some quantity of these products to zero air pollution.

Imposing a tax on pollution has another important consequence: The producer of the product will attempt to lower the tax by devising methods to reduce pollution. The firm may move to an area where the costs of pollution (hence the tax) are lower, or the firm may innovate in its production process to reduce pollution. The tax creates incentives for producers to lower their production costs, which include the tax.

Imposing a tax directly on pollution is preferable to such indirect methods of controlling pollution as allowing existing firms to continue polluting but not permitting others to enter the market or mandating that all firms use a particular production process to reduce pollution. Such indirect approaches eliminate incentives for producers to search for cheaper ways to reduce pollution.

Based on the example of the external costs of pollution, the role of government seems straightforward: when there are widespread external costs, the government should calculate the size of these costs and assess a tax on each unit of output produced. The purchasers and producers of that product then base their decision of how much to purchase on all the costs and benefits (external as well as private) of that product.

Medical Research

The analysis is similar when applied to external benefits. If a university medical researcher develops a new method of performing open-heart surgery that reduces the mortality rate of that procedure, other surgeons will copy the technique to benefit their own patients. An individual researcher/surgeon cannot declare ownership over all possible uses of that technique. If the individual surgeon were not compensated for all those who would eventually benefit, he or she would not find it feasible or worthwhile to invest time and resources to develop new medical techniques. Similarly, medical researchers would underproduce the discovery of basic scientific knowledge, since they would not be able to charge all those who would eventually benefit from a cure for cancer, heart disease, and so on. Though it would be difficult, the government should attempt to calculate the potential benefits and subsidize medical research. Unless the external benefits are assessed and the costs shared by potential beneficiaries, the costs of producing medical research will exceed the private benefits.

An alternative to offering a subsidy to private firms is to give them "property" rights or ownership over their discoveries, namely patent protection. Patent protection is, however, not possible for all basic research or for new surgical techniques. Unpatented medical research or new drug discoveries can be copied by others who then benefit from the discoveries. Drug companies need incentives to compensate them for risks and investments made in research and development.

Immunization

Another example of external benefits involves protection from contagious diseases. Individuals who decide to be immunized against contagious diseases base their decisions solely on the costs and benefits to themselves of immunization. However, those who are not immunized also benefit by receiving a "free ride": their chances of catching that disease are lowered. If immunization were a private decision, not enough individuals would be immunized. The costs of those immunized should be subsidized by imposing a small tax on those who are not immunized but who also benefit. In this manner, the "right" number of people become immunized. The immunization decision thus encompasses private benefits, external benefits, and the costs of immunization. When "transactions costs" are high, that is, the administrative costs of monitoring, collecting taxes, and subsidizing individuals are substantial, it may be less costly to simply require everyone be immunized against certain diseases.

Subsidies to the Medically Indigent

Externalities are also the rationale for providing subsidies to the medically indigent. If the only way the poor received medical care was through voluntary contributions, many people who did not make such contributions would benefit by knowing that the poor are cared for through the contributions of others. Too little would be provided to the medically indigent since those who do not contribute receive a "free ride"; they benefit without having to pay for that benefit. Government intervention would be appropriate to tax those who benefit by knowing the poor receive medical care.

Government Policies when Externalities Exist

In the examples above, the subsidies and taxes are related to the size of the external benefits and costs. Further, the taxes imposed on products that pollute are to be spent for the benefit of those adversely affected. When there are external benefits, then the subsidies are financed by taxes on those who receive the external benefit. Patents are an attempt to recover the external benefits from research. In each case, there is a matching of taxes and subsidies according to external costs and benefits.

Recognizing how externalities affect the correct rate of output in an industry is useful for understanding what government policies would be appropriate in a number of additional areas. For example, when a motorcyclist has an accident and receives a head injury as a result of not wearing a helmet, if the cyclist does not have insurance or sufficient personal funds, government (society) pays their medical expenses. Fines for not wearing helmets is an attempt to make motorcyclists bear the responsibility for external costs that they would otherwise impose on others. At times, imposing requirements (such as helmet use, immunizations, grade school education) may be the least costly approach for achieving the correct output.

The same analogy can be used to describe those who can afford to buy health insurance but refuse. When they incur catastrophic medical expenses they cannot pay for, they then become a burden on society. Requiring everyone who can afford it to have catastrophic medical coverage is a way of avoiding their imposing external costs on others.

Similarly, drunk drivers frequently impose costs on innocent victims. Penalties, such as jail terms, forfeiture of driver's license, fines, and higher alcohol taxes, have been used in attempts to shift the responsibility for these external costs back to those who drink and drive. One recent study concluded that federal and state alcohol taxes should be increased (from an average of 11 cents to 24 cents a drink) to compensate for the external costs imposed on others by excessive drinkers (Manning et al. 1989).

We should be aware, however, that the externalities argument may be misapplied by some to justify intervention by the government in all markets. For example, if you admire someone's garden, should you be taxed to subsidize the gardener? Should the student who asks a particularly clever question in class be subsidized by a tax on other students? These examples, while simple, illustrate several important points about externalities. First, when only a few individuals are involved, the parties concerned should be able to reach an accommodation among themselves without resorting to government intervention. Second, even when there is clear ownership to the property, high transactions costs may make it too costly to charge for external benefits or costs. The owner of the garden can decide whether it is worthwhile to erect a fence and charge a viewing fee. Chances are, the cost of doing so will exceed the amount others are willing to pay. Many may thus receive external benefits simply because excluding them or collecting from them is too costly. Only when the external benefits (or costs) become sufficiently large relative to their transactions costs does it pay for the provider of external benefits either to exclude others or to charge them for their benefits.

A third point the examples above illustrate concerns the relative size of private benefits compared to external benefits. Would the output of the gardener be too small if neighbors did not contribute? Although many goods and services provide external benefits to others, excluding these external benefits does not result in too small a rate of output. In markets where the external benefits are sufficiently small relative to the total private benefits, excluding external benefits does not affect the optimal rate of output. This type of externality, referred to as "inframarginal" externalities, occurs within the market. Thus, gardeners may receive so much pleasure from their gardens that they put forth the same level of effort with or without their neighbors' admiration.

The concept of inframarginal benefit is important to understanding the issue of financing education for health professionals. We all benefit from knowing that we have access to physicians, dentists, and nurses if we become ill. However, if their education were not subsidized, would "too few" physicians be available? The education of physicians is heavily subsidized. The average four-year subsidy for a medical education exceeds $100,000. One reason this cost is so high is that medical schools have little incentive for reducing those costs. For example, some medical educators claim medical students could be admitted to medical school after two years of college, medical education could be reduced by at least one year, the residency period could also be reduced, and innovations in teaching methods and curriculum could reduce the cost still more.

Even if physicians had to pay their entire educational costs themselves, however, the economic return on the costs of becoming a physician has been estimated to be sufficiently attractive that we would have had no less than the current number of physicians. Over time, these economic returns to a medical (and dental) education have changed and varied according to specialty status; they were higher in the 1950–1970s than they are currently. Thus the concept of external benefits in the number of physicians is more likely a case of inframarginal benefits; there have been sufficient private benefits to individuals from becoming a physician to ensure a sufficient supply of physicians even if no subsidies had been provided.

A separate issue is whether individuals with low incomes could afford medical educations if subsidies were removed. Making medical and dental education affordable to all qualified individuals could be accomplished more efficiently by targeting subsidies and loan programs than by subsidizing everyone who attends medical school by the same amount, regardless of income level. The rationale for large educational subsidies for a health professional education should be reexamined.

The Divergence between Theoretical
and Actual Government Policy

Correcting for external costs and benefits creates winners and losers. Taxes and subsidies have redistributive effects; taxpayers have lowered incomes, while subsidy recipients have increased incomes. Every group affected by external costs and benefits desires favorable treatment and has incentives to influence government policy. For example, an industry that pollutes the air and water has a concentrated interest in forestalling government policy that would increase its production costs. All who benefit from environmental protection must organize and provide legislators with political support if anything more than symbolic legislation is to be directed at imposing external costs on those who pollute. The growth of the environmental movement was an attempt to offset the imbalance between those with concentrated (polluters) and diffuse (the public) costs.

The Clean Air Act (1977 Amendments) is illustrative of the divergence between the theoretical approach for resolving external costs and the real-world phenomenon of concentrated and diffuse interests. A greater amount of air pollution is caused when electric utilities burn high-sulfur, rather than low-sulfur, coal. Imposing a tax on the amount of sulfur dioxides (air pollution) emitted would shift the external costs of air pollution to the electric utilities, who would then have an incentive to search for ways to reduce this tax, and consequently the amount of air pollution. One alternative would be for the utilities to switch to low-sulfur coal.

Low-sulfur coal, however, is produced only in the West, and it is cheaper to mine than high-sulfur coal. It is therefore a competitive threat to the Eastern coal interests that produce high-sulfur coal. Faced with taxes based on the amount of air pollution emitted, Midwestern and Eastern utilities would find it cheaper to pay added transportation costs to have low-sulfur coal shipped from the West. However, the concentrated interests of the Eastern coal mines, their heavily unionized employees, and the Senate majority leader (who was from West Virginia, which would have been adversely affected) were able to have legislation passed directed toward the process of reducing pollution rather than directed at the amount of pollution emitted. Requiring utilities merely to use specified technology ("scrubbers") for reducing pollution eliminated the utilities' incentives to use low-sulfur coal. When specific technology is mandated, the utility loses its incentive to maintain that technology in good operating condition and to search for more efficient approaches to reducing pollution. Western utilities that use low-sulfur coal bear the higher costs of using mandated technology even though they could achieve the desired outcomes by less-expensive means (Feldstein 1988).

Summary

Even if medical care markets were competitive, the "right" output might not occur because of external costs and benefits. With regard to personal medical services, externalities are likely to exist related to medical services for the poor and for those who can afford medical insurance but who refuse to purchase coverage for catastrophic illness/injury. And why should medical and dental education be so heavily subsidized? Any external benefits are likely to be "inframarginal," thereby not affecting the number of health professionals. Imposing taxes on personal behaviors (products), such as excessive alcohol consumption, that may result in external costs will also serve as an incentive to reduce these external costs. Most externalities in health care derive from medical research and pollution.

Implicit in discussions of externalities is that government regulation can correct these failures of a competitive market. Politicians, however, may at times be even less responsive to correcting external costs and benefits than producers and consumers. When there are externalities, a theoretical framework for determining appropriate government policy provides a basis for evaluating alternative policies. The divergence between theoretical and actual policies often can be explained by a comparison of the amounts of political support offered by those with concentrated and diffuse interests.

References

Feldstein, P. J. *The Politics of Health Legislation: An Economic Perspective.* Ann Arbor, MI: Health Administration Press, 1988.
Manning, W. G., E. Keeler, J. P. Newhouse, E. Sloss, and J. Wasserman. "The Taxes of Sin: Do Smokers and Drinkers Pay Their Way?" *Journal of the American Medical Association* 261 (17 March 1989): 1604–9.

24

The Canadian Health Care System

The Canadian health care system, also referred to as a *single-payer system*, has been suggested as a model for this country. Starting in the late 1960s, the federal government established the basic guidelines for the system and each province was provided with matching funds, which were contingent on their adherence to the federal guidelines. Under these guidelines, everyone has access to hospital and medical services, and they do not have to pay any deductibles or copayments. Patients have free choice of physician and hospital. Private health insurance is not permitted for these basic hospital and medical services.

Each province sets its own overall health budget and negotiates a total budget with each hospital; the province also negotiates uniform fees with all physicians, who are paid fee-for-service, and who must accept the province's fee as payment in full for their service. Since each province finances its services through an income tax, receives federal matching funds, and pays all medical bills, the need for insurance companies is eliminated. The province controls the adoption and financing of high-technology equipment.

According to its proponents, the Canadian system offers universal coverage, comprehensive hospital and medical benefits, no out-of-pocket expense, and lower administrative costs, while devoting a smaller percent of its GNP to health care and spending less per capita. Would the United States be better off if we were to adopt the Canadian single-payer health system?

Administrative Costs

Advocates of the Canadian system claim that if the United States adopted the Canadian system, it could greatly reduce its administrative costs, thereby financing universal access at no additional cost (Woolhandler and Himmelstein 1991). Many would agree that administrative costs in the United States could be somewhat lowered with standardization of claims processing and billing. However, reducing administrative costs produces a one-time savings, while increased access to all the uninsured is an ongoing expense. More importantly, simple comparisons of administrative expenses between the two countries are misleading.[1]

Administrative and marketing costs could be reduced if the United States were willing to eliminate choice of health plans and agree to a standardized set of health benefits. The United States has a wide variety of health plans, such as HMOs, PPOs, and managed care plans, offering different benefits, with different cost-sharing levels. Under a Canadian system these differences do not exist. The diversity of insurance plans, however, reflects differences in subscribers' preferences and how much they are willing to pay for those preferences. Many people are apparently willing to pay higher administrative costs, hence a higher premium, to be able to have greater choice of health plans.

Lower administrative costs are not synonymous with greater system efficiency. One can imagine very low administrative costs in a system where physicians send their bills to the government and the government simply pays them. These lower administrative costs cause *higher* health care expenditures because they do not detect nor deter inappropriate use or overuse of services. There is a trade-off between having lower administrative costs versus higher health expenditures due to insufficient monitoring of physician behavior. Studies have shown that cost-containment approaches, such as preauthorization for hospital admissions, utilization review for hospitalized patients, catastrophic case management, and physician profiling for appropriateness of care, save money.

The health insurance industry in the United States is very competitive and would only increase administrative costs if the benefits from doing so exceeded their costs. Any savings in administrative costs by eliminating cost-containment techniques and patient cost-sharing would be more than offset by the increased utilization that would occur. The Canadian system is forgoing substantial savings by *not* increasing its administrative costs, investing more in cost-containment programs, and developing monitoring mechanisms of physicians' practice patterns. Canadian physicians have less interference in their practice than do U.S. physicians in managed care organizations.

Limiting Use of Services

Two approaches for limiting use of services whose value is worth less than their costs of production are cost-containment techniques and requiring patients to wait longer. Cost containment is included as an explicit administrative expense, while the implicit patient waiting cost is not.

Expenditure Limits on Health Providers

The basic cost control mechanism used in Canada is expenditure limits on health providers. Hospitals receive an overall budget that they cannot exceed and physicians' fees are negotiated between the government and the medical association. In some Canadian provinces, physicians' incomes are also subject to controls; once physicians' revenues exceed a certain level, then further billings are paid at 25 percent of their fee schedule. Although providers complain about their revenues, and occasionally physicians go on strike, it is claimed that these cost-containment measures have limited the increase in Canadian health expenditures.

Government expenditure limits are the inevitable consequence of having an unlimited demand for medical services. No government can fund the amount that is demanded at zero price. These expenditure limits invariably result in high time costs being imposed on patients; physicians spend less time per visit and the volume of physician visits increase. The physician will have the patient return for multiple short visits rather than provide the services previously provided in one visit. Patient time costs are therefore higher under a "free" system with tight fee controls because each visit requires the same patient travel and waiting time regardless of the length of the visit.

Annual hospital budgets provide administrators with an incentive to fill a portion of their beds with elderly patients staying many days. If they admitted more surgical patients, they would not receive additional funds to purchase the necessary supplies and nursing personnel to serve them. Thus, as inflation diminishes the real value of their budget with which to purchase resources, hospitals admit less acutely ill patients and prolong their stay.

Patient Waiting Times

According to a U.S. Government Accounting Office report on the Canadian health care system, Canadian patients classified as "urgent," meaning the patient has a serious medical condition for which he or she must be monitored and treated while in the hospital, had to wait up to 30 days for an MRI, 30 days for cardiovascular surgery, and 1 year for lithotripsy. If the patient was classified as "elective" (the patient needs to be treated but is not in imminent danger), the waiting times for each of the above needs are up to 16 months, 6 months, and 2 years (U.S. General Accounting Office 1991, 55). There have been reports of patients who have died waiting for heart surgery. In some provinces an aged patient must wait up to 4 years for a hip or knee replacement. The long waits for first-time mammograms virtually eliminates this screening mechanism as a preventive method.

Acknowledging these long waits and its adverse effects on patients, at least two Canadian provinces pay for heart surgery in the United States. About 10 percent of all British Columbians requiring radiation oncology treatment have been sent by the Canadian government to the United States, which is Canada's safety valve. Ontario contracts with hospitals in Buffalo and Detroit for MRI services.

The failure to consider the higher patient time costs in the Canadian system understates health expenditures in Canada. As demand for services exceeds the available supply, many people would be willing to pay more rather than incur the cost of multiple trips, waiting, or doing without. Unfortunately, the Canadian system prohibits the purchase of private health insurance for hospital and medical services. Thus people are legally prohibited from insuring against the risks of not receiving timely care when they require it.

An important consequence of these long waits for medical service is that patients

> . . . experience pain and discomfort, and some may develop psychological problems . . . The condition of some patients may worsen, making surgery more risky . . . because of the long queue for lithotripsy treatment, many doctors perform surgery to remove kidney stones (also resulting in higher costs), putting the patient at higher risk than with a lithotripsy procedure . . . Often patients experience a financial setback, such as decreased income or loss of a job (while waiting in queues) . . . patients are unable to work because they are physically immobile while they wait for a hip or other joint replacement (U.S. General Accounting Office 1991, 59).

Those who are wealthy can afford to skip the queues and purchase medical services in the United States, as did the premier of Quebec.

Technological Innovation

One of the distinguishing features of the U.S. medical system is the rapid rate of technological innovation. Major advances in diagnostic and treatment procedures have occurred. Low-birthweight babies are more likely to survive, and the number and types of organ transplants are increasing. There has been a large shift from inpatient to outpatient surgery, and home infusion therapy is further reducing the use of the hospital. Any comparison of Canada and the United States should consider the criteria used to adopt and make available new technology.

Managed care, the direction in which the United States has been moving since the early 1980s, evaluates new technology in two ways. The simplest case is when new technology reduces cost and increases patient satisfaction; examples are outpatient surgery and home care. The managed care system will invest the necessary capital to bring about these technological savings.

The more difficult area to evaluate is when new technology improves medical outcomes but is more costly than existing technology. Whether or not benefit-increasing technology is adopted depends on the value that subscribers place on access to this technology. If a managed care organization decides not to adopt such technology while other managed care organizations do and, as a result, loses subscribers to their competitors, then they may conclude that they would lose fewer subscribers if they adopted the new technology and increased their subscribers' premiums to pay for it. The rate of technology adoption under managed care competition will depend upon how much subscribers are willing to pay.

In Canada, the availability of capital to invest in cost-saving technology is determined by the government, not the hospital. Given their budget constraints, and their reluctance to raise taxes, governments are less likely to provide capital for new technology and for as many units as would firms competing for subscribers. Outpatient diagnostic and surgical services are less available in Canada, thereby denying patients the benefits (and society the cost savings) of such technological improvements. Examples of differences in availability of technology (per million persons) between Canada, the United States, and California (a state where there is a great deal of managed care) are shown in Figure 24.1.

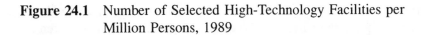

Figure 24.1 Number of Selected High-Technology Facilities per Million Persons, 1989

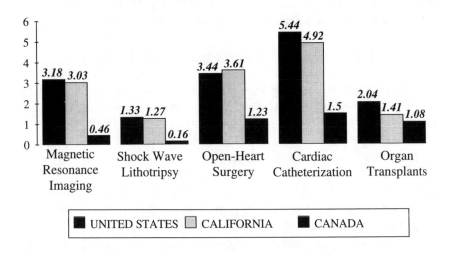

Note: Since 1989 was the latest year for which Canadian data were available, 1989 values were used for all localities to ensure comparability of numbers.

Sources: American Hospital Association (Chicago, IL), *Hospital Statistics, 1990–91*, and the Organization for Economic Cooperation and Development (OECD) (Paris, France).

When a managed care system invests in technology based on its subscribers' willingness to pay, they may adopt technology too soon and have excess technological capacity. Excess capacity, however, means fast access and lower patient risks. Subscribers may be willing to pay higher premiums to have that excess capacity available. If so, then excess technological capacity is appropriate; the benefits to subscribers of that excess capacity is at least equal to their willingness to pay for it. The adoption of new technology under managed care competition would be different from what a government (or quasi-governmental agency) would use, since the government would be concerned with losing political support if it had to raise taxes or incur large budget deficits to increase access to new technology.

Universal Coverage

According to its proponents, there are two major advantages to the Canadian system. The first is universal coverage. However, since adoption of the Canadian system is but one proposal for reform, it should be compared, not to the current U.S. system, but to other health care reform proposals to achieve universal coverage. Thus it is not necessary to adopt the Canadian system solely to achieve universal coverage.

Controlling the Rising Costs of Health Care

To many, the real attractiveness of the Canadian system is based on its presumed ability to control the rising costs of health care. The oft-cited measure of the cost-containment success of the Canadian system is the smaller percent of Canada's GNP devoted to health care. Although correct, this statement is misleading. An important reason for health expenditures being a smaller percent of GNP in Canada has been the faster GNP growth rate in Canada over the past 20 years; inflation-adjusted GNP grew 74 percent in Canada compared to 38 percent in the United States between 1967 and 1987.

A more accurate indication of expenditure growth rates between the two countries is a comparison of the rise in per capita health expenditures. Again one must be careful in making such comparisons since 40 percent of U.S. medical expenditures are by the government for Medicare and Medicaid and in some regions of the United States there is greater reliance on the traditional fee-for-service system than in other regions. This country's system is evolving from one that provided limited, if any, incentives for efficiency until the early 1980s to one in which the private sector, in some states more than others, emphasizes managed care delivery systems. Thus the more recent (from the early 1980s) performance of the U.S. system, particularly in states with a greater portion of their population in managed care, would be more relevant for a comparison with the Canadian system.

As shown in Figure 24.2, between 1980 and 1991 per capita expenditures (not adjusted for inflation) have risen slightly more rapidly in the United States, 9.5 percent per year, than in Canada, 9.2 percent per year. (These annual percent increases in Canada are averaged over years that had wide fluctuations.) When California is included in the comparison, which is heavily reliant on managed care competition, the average annual percent increase in per capita health costs was less than in Canada, only 7.9 percent. (Data on California were only available for the beginning and ending years of 1980–1991.)[2]

Managed care systems in the United States have a financial incentive to use the least-costly combination of medical services. Use of

Figure 24.2   Average Annual Growth in Per Capita Health
Expenditures, 1980–1991

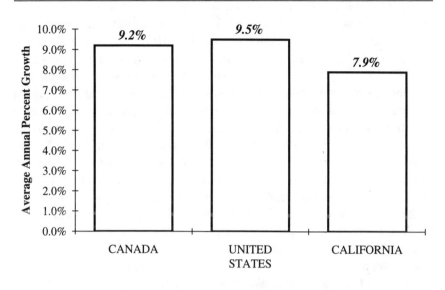

Sources: Health Care Financing Administration (Washington, DC) and the Organization for Economic Cooperation and Development (OECD) (Paris, France).

the hospital is subject to review, outpatient diagnostics and surgery are used whenever possible, and catastrophic case management may involve renovation of the patient's home to make it a lower-cost and more-convenient setting to care for the patient.

The efficiency gains from managed care are evident in a comparison of utilization data between the United States and Canada. The average length of stay in Canadian hospitals is 50 percent greater than in the United States, 10.8 days versus 7.1 days (in California, it is 6.4 days); hospital patient-days per 1,000 population are 63 percent greater than in the United States, 1,550 versus 950 (California has 678 days). The average length of stay for those 65 years and older is very high in Canada since few alternative arrangements are available. Canadian hospitals are used inappropriately; many services could be provided in an outpatient setting, the physician's office, or in the patient's home.

In recent years the rising costs of health care in Canada and a deep recession in the late 1980s have caused the federal government to reduce its matching funds commitment to the provinces. The federal government has decreased its matching funds from 50 percent initially to less than 40 percent, and under the terms of a recently enacted (1991) law, the federal contribution could disappear in ten years. As these federal matching funds are phased out, each province's incentive to comply with the federal guidelines will also decline. The rising cost of the Canadian health system has placed an increasing financial burden on each province.

The consequence of these rising costs on both the federal and provincial governments has been to spend *less* on health care. As shown in Figure 24.3, the annual percent increase in inflation-adjusted per capita health expenditures has fallen dramatically since 1987 (although the average for the period 1980–1991 is just slightly less than in the United States). This recent dramatic decline is due to government budgetary problems and not to new cost-containment approaches. In the past when such large declines occurred, such as in the early and late 1970s, it was followed by sharp increases in following years. Because of the Canadian recession and federal and provincial budgetary constraints, however, it may be difficult to make up for these sharp declines in financing. Two outcomes would then be likely: increasing shortages of medical services and technology and/or changes in how Canada's health care system is financed, such as the imposition of deductibles, copayments, and premiums. We are likely to observe Canada moving away from the type of health system that single-payer advocates are proposing for the United States.

Should the United States Adopt the Canadian System?

Why would the United States move to a health care system in which there are serious problems of access to care and to technology and more rapidly increasing per capita health care costs than California, a state with a comparable population but reliant on managed care?

According to various surveys, Canadians are more pleased with their health system than are Americans. But it is important to keep in mind that Canadians share a set of egalitarian values with respect to access to care in their health system that are not shared by a majority of Americans. These differences in values are important to the acceptance of the Canadian, or single-payer, system for the United States.

Before the United States selects another country's medical system, it should be clear both as to the accuracy of the statements that are being made about the performance of that country's medical system and the

Figure 24.3   Annual Percent Growth in Real Per Capita Health
Expenditures in Canada and the United States,
1965–1991

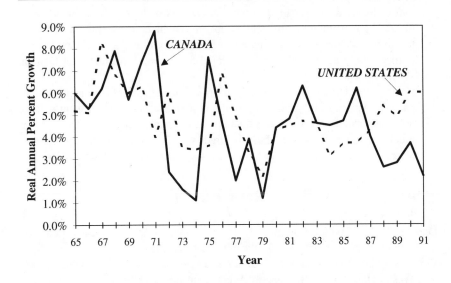

Note: Values adjusted for inflation using the price index for gross domestic product
for each country.
Source: Organization for Economic Cooperation and Development (Paris, France),
OECD Health Systems, Volumes I and II, 1993.

criteria by which a system should be evaluated. The percent of GNP
devoted to medical care should not be the overriding objective of a medical system, otherwise we should use the British National Health Service,
which performs better on this criterion, but is clearly unacceptable on
other grounds. Incentives for efficiency and innovation, access to medical
technology based on subscribers' willingness to pay, and adequate funding for those with low incomes are more appropriate criteria. Reliance
on competitive managed care systems, with vouchers for those with low
incomes, is more likely to achieve these performance criteria.

Notes

1. The administrative savings of moving to a Canadian system are believed to
   be grossly overstated. For example, in calculating administrative savings,

the expense of administering self-insured employer plans was included in the expense ratio of insurers. However, the claims payments made on behalf of self-insured employers were not included as part of the insurers' premiums, thereby falsely inflating the expense ratio. Further, included as part of insurers' overhead are premium taxes (which are a transfer payment to state governments), investment income (which is essentially a return to employers for advance payment of premiums), and a return on capital (which would also have to be calculated for a public insurer). See Danzon 1992.

2. Canada, the United States, and California are not, of course, strictly comparable. Although the uninsured in the United States and California receive uncompensated care from physicians and hospitals, they do not receive as much care as if they were fully insured, which would lead to a somewhat lower rate of increase in the United States and California than in Canada.

References

Danzon, P. M. "Hidden Overhead Costs: Is Canada's System Really Less Expensive?" *Health Affairs* 11 (Spring 1992): 21–43.

U.S. General Accounting Office. *Canadian Health Insurance.* GAO/HRD-91-90. Washington, DC: U.S. General Accounting Office, 1991.

Woolhandler, S., and D. Himmelstein. "The Deteriorating Administrative Efficiency of the U.S. Health Care System." *The New England Journal of Medicine* 324 (2 May 1991): 1253–58.

25

Employer-Mandated
National Health Insurance

President Clinton has proposed, as part of his national health insurance proposal, that employers be required to provide health insurance to their employees and dependents. An employer mandate has a great deal of political support. The Pepper Commission, named after its late chairman, Claude Pepper, endorsed this approach toward national health insurance; Hawaii has instituted it; and a number of other states are considering it. The AMA also favors it as a way to finance health care for the working uninsured.

Approximately 37 million people under age 65 are uninsured, and about two-thirds of them are either employed or in a family with an employed member. Therefore mandating employers to provide their employees with health insurance would cover a large percent of the uninsured, at small cost to the government. If employers chose not to provide health insurance to their employees, then they would have to pay a new payroll tax (either a fixed amount per employee or a percentage of payroll) into a state pool for the uninsured—hence the name, "play or pay" national health insurance.

Although there are variations on the basic approach, mandated employer proposals generally require the employer to pay 80 percent and the employee 20 percent of the cost of the insurance. Employees working part-time would be eligible for the employer's health insurance. "Play or pay" proposals generally mandate that all employers with more than 100 employees be required to immediately participate; firms with fewer employees would have to participate in subsequent years. The transition of smaller firms, under some proposals, might be eased by providing the firm with a tax credit to offset the firm's higher costs.

Before analyzing the consequences of mandating employers to provide health insurance to the working uninsured, it is useful to examine who the uninsured are and why they do not have insurance.

The Uninsured

Of the 215 million persons who were less than 65 in 1990 (those who are 65 years of age are eligible for Medicare), about 17 percent, or 37 million, were without private health insurance. As shown in Figure 25.1, 25 percent of the uninsured are under the age of 18; 18 percent are between the ages 18 and 24; 23 percent are between 25 and 34 years of age; and the highest percent of the uninsured, 34 percent, are between the ages 35 and 64.

Figure 25.1 Percent Distribution of the Uninsured Population by Age Group

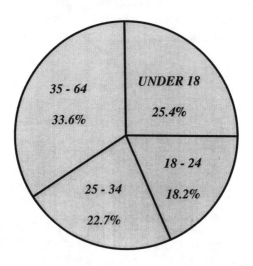

Note: Figures are based on the analysis of data from the U.S. Census Bureau's 1993 Current Population Survey.

Source: Employee Benefit Research Institute (EBRI), *Issue Brief #145*, January 1994.

Although Whites represent 61 percent of the total number of uninsured, uninsured Whites represent a smaller portion of all Whites (14 percent) than do uninsured Blacks as a percent of all Blacks (24 percent). Hispanics have the highest uninsured percentage, 33 percent. Regionally, most of the uninsured are in the South, 41 percent. The West is second with 25 percent; the Midwest has 19 percent; and the Northeast has the fewest, 15 percent.

An important characteristic of the employed uninsured is the size of the firm in which they work. The fewer the number of employees, the greater is the likelihood that the employer does not provide health insurance. Thus 25 percent of employees in small firms (under 25 employees) are uninsured, compared to only 7 percent in large firms (over 1,000 employees). As a percent of all the employed uninsured, 51 percent are in firms with less than 25 employees and 14 percent are in firms with 25–99 employees. Thus 65 percent of the total number of employed uninsured are in firms with fewer than 100 employees (see Table 25.1).

A second important work-related characteristic of the employed uninsured is their low wages. As shown in Table 25.2, as of 1991, 52 percent of the employed uninsured earned less than $6 an hour; another 29 percent earned between $6 and $10 per hour. Thus 81 percent earned

Table 25.1   Uninsured Workers under 65 by Size of Firm, 1990

Size of Firm (Number of Employees)	Number of Workers (Millions)	Number of Uninsured Workers (Millions)	Number of Uninsured Workers as Percentage of Total Uninsured Workers	Percentage of People in Group Who Are Uninsured
Under 25	32.9	8.2	51.1	25.0
25 to 99	14.9	2.4	14.0	16.2
100 to 499	16.0	1.8	11.2	11.3
500 to 999	6.5	0.5	3.1	7.7
1,000 and over	43.5	3.2	19.7	7.3
All firms	113.7	16.1	100.0	14.2

Source: Congressional Budget Office, *Rising Health Care Costs*, April 1991, Tables B-5 and B-6, pp. 73–74.

less than $10 per hour. Only 6.5 percent of uninsured employees earned more than $15 per hour.

Why the Uninsured Do Not Have Health Insurance

There are two important reasons why the employed uninsured are less likely to have health insurance. The first is that the price of insurance is higher (consequently the demand is lower) for those who are employed in small firms. There are three reasons for this higher price. Smaller firms are unable to take advantage of economies in administering and marketing health insurance, thereby resulting in higher insurance costs per employee. Insurance companies also charge higher premiums in small firms to make allowance for adverse selection, believing that many employees will join just to take advantage of health benefits. Or, for example, an owner might hire a sick relative so the medical costs can be paid. In larger firms, with lower turnover rates, it is less likely that employment is primarily for the purpose of receiving health benefits. And finally, many states have mandated various benefits, such as in vitro fertilization and hair transplants, that must be included in any health insurance plan sold in their state. Once included in the insurance policy, employees use these services, thereby increasing the insurance premium. Larger firms, however, are able to self-insure, thereby becoming exempt from the costs of these additional mandates. Smaller firms are too small to self-insure; they therefore have to pay the higher premium, which lessens their demand for health insurance.

The second reason for the lower demand for health insurance in small firms is the low incomes of their employees. Since 52 percent of the employed uninsured earn less than $6 per hour, health insurance

Table 25.2   Percent Distribution of Uninsured Workers by Wage Rate, 1991

Hourly Wage Rate	Percent of Uninsured
$5.99 or less	51.8%
$6.00–9.99	29.0
$10.00–14.99	12.7
$15.00 or more	6.5

Source: K. R. Levit, G. L. Olin, and S. W. Letsch, "Americans' Health Insurance Coverage, 1980–91," *Health Care Financing Review* 14 (Fall 1992): 54.

premiums would result in a major reduction in their funds available for other necessities. When these low-wage employees or their families become ill, they are likely to become eligible for Medicaid, which is their health insurance plan.

Consequences of Employer-Mandated Health Insurance

Nonuniversal Coverage

Employer-mandated health insurance by itself cannot achieve universal coverage. Even if all the working uninsured were covered by an employer mandate, those employed part-time and those not employed, together with their dependents, would still not have insurance coverage. This would leave approximately one-third of the uninsured without coverage. To achieve universal coverage, an employer mandate must be combined with an insurance subsidy program for these other population groups.

Inequities for Low-Income Employees

Advocates of an employer mandate have proposed that small firms be given tax credits or subsidies to induce them to offer health insurance to their employees. This approach, however, is likely to be inequitable. While many low-wage employees work in small firms, not everyone employed by small firms earns a low income, such as small legal firms or physician groups. The subsidy could be limited to those small firms with low average incomes. However, there are low-wage employees in large firms who would not receive subsidies. To eliminate these inequities, tax subsidies should be targeted to those in need and not according to the size of firm.

Who Pays for Employer Mandates?

Employer mandates require the employer to pay 80 percent and the employee 20 percent of the cost of health insurance. Thus it would appear that most of the cost will be borne by the firm. However, whether the employer or the employee actually bears the burden of the tax, does not depend upon whom the tax is imposed. In competitive industries, firms do not make excess profits; otherwise, other firms (including foreign firms) would enter that industry until excess profits no longer exist. When employers are earning a competitive rate of return, they will be unable to bear the burden of the additional tax themselves—they would eventually go out of business. Instead, faced with a new employee tax, employers will, within a short period, shift the cost of that tax to others by increasing the prices they charge, decreasing the cash wages paid to their employees, or both.

Imposing a per employee tax on the employer is likely to result in one of three possible outcomes. Exactly which combination occurs will depend on the particular labor and product markets in which the firm competes, since the nature of these markets will determine how much of the higher labor costs are shifted back onto the employee and how much gets shifted forward in the form of higher consumer prices. First, to the extent that employees are flexible between the relative portions of their total compensation that goes to cash wages and fringe benefits (including health insurance), then the cost of labor to the employer is unchanged. An increased employer tax to pay for their employees' insurance would result in lower wages, thereby not increasing the cost of labor to the firm. Although employees receive more health insurance, they clearly value the health insurance less than the cash wages it takes to purchase it, since they could have purchased the insurance previously but chose not to. Thus the first effect is to make uninsured low-wage employees worse off by forcing a change in how they spend their limited incomes.

It is unlikely, however, that the employee tax can be shifted entirely back to the employee in the form of lower cash wages. Many employees are at or near the minimum wage; these minimum wage laws prevent the transferring of the health insurance costs to the employee because they cannot receive lower cash wages. Further, the mix between wages and health insurance is not perfectly flexible, particularly right away; therefore the cost of labor to the firm will be increased. With higher labor costs, the firm will have to increase the prices of its goods and services. These increased prices in turn will lead consumers to purchase fewer goods and services. With a smaller demand for its output, the firm will need fewer employees. The firm will also decrease its demand for labor by decreasing the use of part-time employees (if they must be covered) and increase overtime of full-time employees. Thus a second effect of a health insurance tax per employee is that it raises the cost of these employees and causes fewer of them to be employed.

To the extent that labor costs are increased, then part of the employee tax is shifted forward in the form of higher consumer prices. This third effect of the tax results in a regressive form of consumer taxation because all consumers, regardless of their incomes, pay higher prices. Those higher prices represent a greater portion of the income of low-income consumers than they do for high-income consumers. This is an inequitable method of financing universal health insurance.

Cost to Government

The employer mandate is attractive to government because it shifts the cost of low-wage labor off Medicaid onto the employees and their employers. However, an employer mandate is more costly to the government than it appears. First, since employer-paid health insurance is not considered to be taxable income, the change in compensation from cash wages to health insurance decreases Social Security taxes as well as state and federal income taxes. Second, government welfare expenditures will be higher as a result of the increase in unemployment, which would result from those who are near the minimum wage and when wages are not flexible downward. Third, additional subsidies and taxes would be necessary to finance care for approximately one-third of the uninsured who are not employed or a dependent of an employee if this approach is to achieve universal coverage.

Under "pay or play" proposals, many employers will conclude that it is less costly for them to pay an employee tax rather than provide their employees with health insurance. The average health insurance premium is about $300 a month, or $3600 a year, per employee for family coverage. If an employer has to purchase health insurance for its employees or pay 8 percent of payroll into a government pool, then it would cost less to pay the 8 percent tax for any employee making less than $50,000 a year. As medical costs continue to increase, more employers are likely to opt for the "pay" rather than "play" option. One study estimates that 35 percent of employers currently providing their employees with health insurance would find it cheaper to drop that coverage and pay the tax. As many as 40 million employees and their dependents would lose their coverage and be forced into the government pool (Zedlewski, Acs, and Winterbottom 1992).

If employers have an option to "pay or play," then setting the tax too low will make it less costly for employers to pay an employee tax rather than provide health insurance. The government will discover that it cannot fund the same set of benefits on the 8 percent tax revenue; it has been variously estimated that to fund the minimum benefits the tax would have to be 11–12 percent rather than 8 percent of payroll.

In addition to employees whose benefits previously cost more than the "pay or play" tax, subsidies would also be required for all those who are eligible for the public pool but cannot afford it. There will be insufficient revenues to finance the expanded public pool.

Just as the cost of other health programs, such as Medicare Part A and Part B, increased beyond initial expectations, the necessary tax to finance an employer mandate will have to rise beyond the 8 percent level. And as the number of employees (particularly low-wage employees) in the government pool increases, the government will be faced with the choice of either raising taxes or limiting payments to hospitals and physicians. The result is likely to be a very large Medicaid program for the increasing number of employees shifted to the government pool.

If all firms are required (as under the Clinton administration proposal) to pay a specified percent of payroll as a tax, then the employer's liability for their employees' medical expenses is limited to the size of that percentage tax. The employer no longer has an incentive to use innovative cost-containment measures. The responsibility for managing the medical expenses for all those in the public pool falls to the managers of the pool, rather than to each employer, to be concerned with their own employees' medical expenses.

Financing national health insurance through an employer mandate relies on a hidden and an inequitable method of financing health insurance for the uninsured. By imposing the tax on the employer it is made to appear as though the employer bears the cost of the tax. The tax, however, is shifted both to consumers and to employees. In both cases, it is a regressive tax. When the tax is borne by labor in the form of lower cash wages, low-wage employees have to pay a higher percent of their incomes for health insurance. The portion of the tax borne by low-wage consumers represents a higher portion of their income.

And one of the major concerns with an employer mandate is its effect on the firm's demand for labor. As the cost of labor increases, the demand for labor will decrease. The job loss, particularly among those employees near the minimum wage whose wages cannot be reduced to offset the employer tax, is estimated to be 3 million.

This hidden tax on consumers and employees also understates its budgetary effects on the government. Federal and state governments lose tax revenues.

Given the inequities and inefficiencies associated with an employer mandate, why has it received so much political support?

Political Advantages of
Employer-Mandated Health Insurance

The political advantages received by various interest groups outweigh the inequities and inefficiencies that an employer mandate imposes on others. Congress would not have to raise a large amount of tax revenues for an employer-mandated national health insurance plan; it would even reduce Medicaid expenditures. Thus it offers the illusion that federal expenditures are little affected. States, whose Medicaid expenditures are increasing faster than any other state expenditure, are facing deficits and are reluctant to raise taxes. If the states are able to shift the medical costs of low-wage employees and their dependents from Medicaid onto the employees and their employers, it would alleviate the state's own fiscal problems. Hospital and physician organizations favor this approach because it would provide insurance to those previously without it, thereby increasing the demand for hospital and physician services. Payment levels to health providers would be higher than Medicaid payment levels. Health insurance companies would similarly benefit since the demand for their services would increase.

Large employers and their unions, who would be unaffected since they already provide health benefits in excess of the mandated minimum, believe they will benefit competitively from mandated employer insurance. Large firms with high labor costs would like to increase the costs of their low-wage competitors, thereby making them less price competitive. Robert Crandall, the chair of American Airlines, stated that as a result of the difference in their employees' medical costs and those of Continental Airlines, "Continental's unit cost advantage vs. American's is enormous—and worse yet, is growing! . . . which is why we're supporting . . . legislation mandating minimum (health) benefit levels for all employees" (*Wall Street Journal* 1987).

Under the Clinton administration's employer mandate proposal, no employer would have to pay more than 8 percent of payroll for its employees' health care. The automobile companies and their unions would be large beneficiaries under this proposal. Health expenses for auto employees are currently in excess of 15 percent of payroll. Thus these companies and their employees would presumably receive the same benefits for less and be able to have higher cash wages. Who will be paying the higher taxes to make this possible?

Political Opposition to Employer-Mandated Health Insurance

The major political opposition to an employer mandate has been by small business. They are aware of the consequences of an employee tax on the prices they would have to charge, on the demand for their goods and services, and on their demand for labor. The opposition by small business is the major reason why this legislation has not been enacted in many states where it has been proposed. Before this type of legislation can be enacted, the political opposition by small firms will have to be bought off, either by exempting them from the legislation or by offsetting their higher costs by providing them with a subsidy.

References

Wall Street Journal. "Notable & Quotable." (8 August 1987): 16.
Zedlewski, S., G. Acs, and C. Winterbottom. "Play-or-Pay Employer Mandates: Potential Effects." *Health Affairs* 11 (Spring 1992): 62–83.

26

National Health Insurance: Which Approach and Why?

National health insurance (NHI) is an idea whose time has come, and then gone, and is now once again on the political horizon. A variety of national health insurance plans have been proposed, from replicating the Canadian system, to mandating employers to provide coverage for their employees, to providing tax credits for the purchase of health insurance. The proponents of each of these approaches claim different virtues for their plan—one plan is more likely to limit the rise in medical expenditures, another will require a smaller tax increase to implement, and still another may be more politically acceptable. Unless there are some commonly accepted criteria as to what NHI should accomplish, it becomes difficult to evaluate and choose among these plans.

Criteria for National Health Insurance

Production Efficiency

Economists are concerned with two issues: efficiency and equity. Efficiency has two parts. The first is *production efficiency*—are the services (for a given level of quality) produced at the lowest cost? Efficiency in production not only includes whether the hospital portion of a treatment is produced at lowest-cost but also whether the treatment itself is produced at minimum cost. Unless the treatment is provided in the lowest-cost mix of settings, such as hospitals, outpatient care, and home care, the overall cost of providing the treatment will not be as low as is possible. To ensure that each component of the treatment (such as hospital services), as well as the entire medical treatment, is produced efficiently, the providers of medical services require appropriate incentives. This first criterion for judging proposed NHI plans—namely, whether the plan includes appropriate incentives for efficiency in production—is not controversial.

Efficiency in Consumption

The second aspect of efficiency, referred to as *efficiency in consumption*, is controversial. In other sectors of the economy consumers make choices regarding the amount of their income they allocate to different goods and services. Consumers have incentives to consider both the costs as well as the benefits of their choices. Spending their funds on one good means forgoing the benefits of another good or service. When consumers allocate their funds in this manner, resources are directed to their highest-valued uses, as perceived by consumers.

There are some who are opposed to having the consumer decide how much should be spent on medical services; they would prefer to have the government decide how much is allocated to medical care, as in the Canadian system. Canadians are unable to purchase additional private health insurance to forgo waits for open-heart surgery or treatment of other illnesses. Inherent in the concept of efficiency in consumption is that the purpose of national health insurance is to benefit the consumer and that the consumer will be free to purchase more medical services than the minimum level offered in any health insurance plan.

Even if one accepts the concept of consumer decision making, there is a concern that the costs of the consumers' choices are distorted. If the cost of one choice is subsidized while other choices are not, then consumers will demand more of the subsidized choice than if they had to pay its full costs, resulting in inefficiency in consumption. For example, employer-purchased health insurance is not considered by the government to be taxable income to the employee. Consumers therefore purchase more health insurance since health insurance is paid with before-tax dollars while other choices, such as housing, must be paid with after-tax dollars. The tax-free status of employer-paid health insurance is therefore a cause of inefficiency because the costs of the consumers' other choices are in after-tax dollars.

Thus a second criterion for NHI plans is whether consumers are able to decide how much of their incomes they want to spend on medical services and whether there are any subsidies that distort the costs of their choices.

Equity

When NHI plans are evaluated on how those with low incomes are to be subsidized, it is necessary to examine which population groups benefit (are subsidized) and which population groups bear the costs (pay higher taxes). For example, if long-term care is provided to all the aged and financed by a sales tax, all the aged receive some benefits and everyone would contribute to its financing. For equitable redistribution to occur, those with higher incomes are expected to incur net costs (their taxes are in excess of their benefits) while those with low incomes should receive net benefits (benefits in excess of costs). Whenever an individual's costs are not equal to the benefits they receive, redistribution occurs. Since the objective of national health insurance is presumably to provide medical care to the poor, high-income groups should subsidize the care of those with lower incomes; whether this occurs is the third criterion for evaluating alternative NHI plans.

Crucial for determining whether or not redistribution goes from high- to low-income groups is the definition of beneficiaries and how the plan is financed. Ideally, those with lowest incomes should receive the largest subsidy (which would decline as income rises), and the subsidy should be financed by a tax that is either proportional or progressive to income. If the tax is proportional to income (e.g., 5 percent), then those with lowest incomes would receive a net benefit, since the subsidy they receive (sufficient to purchase a minimum benefit package) exceeds the taxes they pay. When a progressive tax, such as an income tax, is used to finance benefits to those with low incomes, then the redistribution from those with high incomes to those with low incomes is even greater.

A regressive tax, such as a payroll or sales tax, will take a higher portion of income from a low-income employee than from a high-income employee and is therefore a less-desirable method of financing redistributive programs. In fact, when a regressive tax is used, the tax paid by many low-income persons may exceed the value of the benefits they receive. For example, if everyone is eligible to receive the same set of benefits, but those with higher incomes use more medical services, perhaps because they are located closer to medical providers or their attitudes toward seeking care are different from those with less education (who also have low income), then the taxes paid by those with low incomes may exceed the benefits they receive. Perversely, those with low incomes may end up subsidizing the care received by those with higher incomes. It is important to examine the size of the benefits received, by income level, in relation to the amount of tax paid. Income tax financing is the preferred way to achieve redistribution since it results in greater net benefits to those with low incomes.

Based on the above discussion of efficiency and equity, an NHI plan should provide incentives for efficiency in production, enable consumers to decide how much of their incomes they want to spend on medical care, and be redistributive—those with lower incomes receive net benefits while those with higher incomes bear costs in excess of their benefits. All NHI proposals should be judged by how well they fulfill these criteria. An important reason why NHI plans fail to meet these criteria is that they have objectives other than improving efficiency or equity; these other objectives thus become obvious when the efficiency and redistributive criteria are used. The following proposal for national health insurance achieves both the equity and efficiency criteria (for a more complete description of this plan, see Pauly et al. 1991).

An Efficient and Equitable Proposal for National Health Insurance

Mandatory Minimum Levels of Health Insurance

To achieve universal coverage the government must ensure that the two groups without insurance—those who can afford insurance but refuse to purchase it and those who cannot afford insurance—are covered by any NHI plan. To do so, the federal government should, first, require everyone to have a minimum level of health insurance. The reason for requiring universal coverage is to ensure that those who become ill do not become a financial burden to others; their costs should not be shifted to those with insurance or require taxpayers to pay their medical expenses. Many uninsured are financially able to purchase health insurance but choose not to do so. Further, since the requirement for insurance is on the individual, insurance would be "portable" with the employee as he or she changes jobs. Employers would not be concerned with the health status of new employees.

Subsidies for Low Incomes through Vouchers

Second, those who cannot afford to purchase the minimum amount should receive government assistance. A subsidy should be provided to those with low incomes for the purchase of health insurance from a governmentally approved plan. For those with low incomes, the subsidy would be equal to the premium from a managed care insurer for the minimum level of benefits. Those receiving such a subsidy would be issued a "voucher," which would provide them with membership in a managed care plan. Those with somewhat higher incomes would receive a smaller subsidy; they would be required to pay part of the cost of the health insurance voucher. At some higher level of income, the subsidy would be eliminated.

Differing Levels of Insurance

Everyone would be required to purchase the same core medical services; these might be equivalent to what is offered in a low-cost managed care plan. However, those with higher incomes could have higher cost-sharing provisions. These higher deductibles and copayments up to a maximum stop loss, which would vary according to income, would result in lower insurance premiums. Those with higher incomes can afford to pay larger amounts out-of-pocket without becoming a burden on society. Catastrophic insurance coverage therefore becomes the minimum level of benefits. Since income and ability to pay for medical care varies, a catastrophic policy for lower-income persons would not be the same as a catastrophic policy for those with higher incomes. Thus the definition of a catastrophic policy should be based on income. For example, a family with $50,000 income might have to pay a maximum of $2000 out-of-pocket, while someone with $75,000 income might have to pay 6 percent of their income out-of-pocket.

Operation of the System

The system would be operationalized as follows: When a person files an income tax return he or she would attach proof of purchase of a minimum-benefit insurance policy. The government would allow the person to deduct from his or her tax liability a fixed dollar credit that is equal to the premium of the minimum-benefit insurance policy. If the credit exceeded his or her tax liability, the person would receive a refund for the difference. The tax credit would decline for those with higher incomes and eventually be eliminated at some higher level of income. If a person failed to attach proof of purchase for a minimum health plan, then the government would add the appropriate premium to the person's tax liability and enroll him or her in a managed care plan. For those who do not file income taxes, the local welfare agency would determine their eligibility and provide them with a subsidy for the purchase of health insurance from a qualified health plan. Operationally, they would be issued a voucher for care in a managed care plan. The Medicaid program would no longer be necessary since the income-related subsidy would replace it.

Fallback Insurance

To ensure that everyone would be able to join a health plan, the government would solicit bids from one or more insurers in an area to be the "fallback" insurer. The fallback insurer, which would likely be a managed care plan, would specify the premiums for each minimum policy (the same core services with different cost-sharing limits). The fallback health plan would serve two groups: those who voluntarily join because the premiums are lower than competing health plans and those assigned to it because they did not indicate proof of health plan coverage on their income tax return.

The tax credit that would be used to offset a person's tax liability would be a fixed amount and would be based on the premiums available from the fallback insurer. Requiring the government to accept bids from a fallback insurer will ensure that the government's tax credit is sufficient to enable those with low incomes to purchase the core medical benefits from a private health plan.

Guaranteed Renewability of Coverage

To become a qualified health plan, the health plan would have to offer guaranteed renewability of coverage at standard rates. A separate high-risk pool could be established for those who are currently uninsurable. For example, individuals without health insurance who require open-heart surgery would be able to join the high-risk pool at subsidized premiums. Over time there would be no need for such a risk pool since everyone would have insurance and all insurance plans would have to guarantee renewability at standard rates.

Effect on Employer-Employee Relationship

The proposed NHI plan should have little effect on current employer and employee relationships. Even though the obligation is on the employee and not the employer, employers would continue to act as a purchaser of health insurance for their employees. Employees would prefer that their employers maintain their current role because of administrative economies in being part of a large group. Also, employers would be better able than their employees to evaluate competing health plans. The employer would deduct the employee's premium from wages and include on the employee's W-2 form that the employee has coverage in a qualified plan. More employers are likely to offer health coverage to their employees now that the obligation is on the employee and not on them.

Currently, small employer groups and individuals are charged higher premiums than large employer groups because of higher administrative expense and insurers' fear of adverse selection—that is, that the person wants insurance because he or she is ill. Since everyone would be required to have health insurance, insurance companies would be less concerned about adverse selection. Further, the self-employed and other individuals would always have access to the fallback insurer, whose premiums would reflect the lower administrative costs associated with a large group.

Elimination of State Mandates

With minimum benefit levels there would be no need for state health mandates, such as requiring all insurance plans to include chiropractic services or to cover hair transplants. While some of these state mandates would likely be included in most insurance plans, eliminating the more than 750 state mandates across the 50 states would reduce the cost of health insurance. If individuals wished to purchase these services on their own with after-tax dollars, they would be free to do so.

**Elimination of the Tax Exclusion for
Employer-Purchased Health Insurance**

The tax exclusion for employer-purchased health insurance should also be eliminated. Tax-free health insurance primarily benefits those with the highest incomes. As employer-purchased health insurance becomes part of the employee's taxable income, tax revenues will increase by $60 billion a year, which is equal to what the government is currently losing by not having these fringe benefits taxed. These funds could be used to provide those with low incomes income-related health insurance vouchers. Employees would be permitted to purchase more comprehensive coverage than is provided in the minimum insurance plan. However, since there no longer would be any tax advantages to buying more comprehensive insurance, it is likely that employees will decide to take more of their income in the form of higher salaries and wages. For political reasons, the entire tax subsidy for employer-purchased health insurance may not be eliminated; it could be phased out over time or amounts above a certain limit could be subject to income taxes.

Elimination of Medicare

Over time, the Medicare system could become part of this new NHI plan, since it would be politically difficult to institute an income-related system for those currently on Medicare. Thus current Medicare beneficiaries (and those close to the Medicare eligibility age) would receive a fully subsidized voucher in a managed care plan. Those who are perhaps between the ages of 45 and 60 could receive a partially subsidized voucher related to their Medicare contributions, and the Medicare system could be phased out for those less than 45 years of age.

Advantages of the Proposed Plan

Reliance on a competitive health insurance market and delivery system is more likely to achieve an efficient and high-quality medical system than one that is controlled by the government. Less-comprehensive health insurance, paid for with after-tax dollars, will provide employees with an incentive to be more concerned with their choice of health plan, its premium, and its benefits.

The income-related voucher meets the efficiency and redistribution criteria in the following ways: Everyone is obligated to have a minimum set of health insurance benefits. Those with the lowest incomes would be assured of adequate health insurance and would receive the largest net benefits under the proposed plan. The size of the subsidy would decline as income increases. The tax credits would be financed by a visible and equitable tax. Employer-purchased health insurance (perhaps above a certain dollar amount) would become part of the employee's taxable income. The resulting increased tax revenues, together with funds from the income tax system and from the current Medicaid system, would provide the funding for the income-related subsides. Thus the financing source is based on progressive taxation. And the requirement of universal coverage means that cost shifting by those who do not purchase insurance to those who do will no longer occur.

The mandate to have insurance is on the individual, not on the employer; thus the individual would be able to change jobs without fear of losing insurance or being denied coverage because of a preexisting condition. Since everyone would be required to have insurance, even if a person develops a preexisting condition an employer should be willing to hire that person because there would not be any additional health insurance cost to the employer. Insurers would not be able to cancel a person's coverage and would have to guarantee rate increases within standard rate bands.

Employees would have incentives to make cost-conscious choices, and a competitive health insurance market would be relied on for achieving efficiency and quality. The greater out-of-pocket liability for employees will increase their price sensitivity to different managed care plans. And government contracting with managed care plans to select the fallback insurer will ensure that competition among managed care plans for these contracts will occur, thereby benefiting those enrolled. Price (premium) sensitivity by both employees (and employers acting on their behalf) and the government accepting bids for the fallback insurance plan will provide price incentives for insurers, managed care plans, and providers, such as hospitals and physicians, to be as efficient as possible. Unless health plans are responsive to consumer demands at a premium the consumer is willing to pay, the health plan will not be able to compete in a price-competitive market.

The rate of increase in medical expenditures would be based on what consumers, balancing cost and use of services, decide is appropriate. Arbitrary limits on total medical expenditures would not be established by the government. Instead, the rate of increase in medical expenditures will be the "correct" rate since consumers would decide how much they are willing to spend to achieve additional medical benefits. Consumers, through their choices, will make the trade-offs between access to care and premiums to pay for that level of access. The outcome will be an appropriate rate of increase in medical expenditures.

Reference

Pauly, M., P. Danzon, P. Feldstein, and J. Hoff. "A Plan for 'Responsible National Health Insurance'." *Health Affairs* 10 (Spring 1991): 5–25.

27

Financing Long-Term Care

Spending for long-term care (LTC) services is expected to increase sharply over the next several decades. The population is aging; as shown in Figure 27.1, the number of aged are expected to increase from 30 million (12.5 percent of the population) in 1990 to 65 million (22 percent) in 2030. An aging population, living longer, increases the number at risk for LTC services. While the demand for services to assist the impaired aged in those activities necessary for daily living is increasing, the cost of providing those services is also rising, at a rate faster than general inflation. How these services should be financed, and by whom, is an important public policy dilemma.

The Nature of Long-Term Care

LTC services consist of a range of services for those who are unable to function independently. These include services that can be provided in the person's home, such as shopping, preparing meals, and housekeeping services; in community-based facilities, such as adult day care; and in nursing homes for those who are unable to perform most of the activities necessary for daily living, such as bathing, toileting, dressing, and so on. The nursing home is but the end of a spectrum in which all of the basic activities are available for those with the most physical and mental impairments.

The need for LTC increases with age. As shown in Table 27.1, the greatest needs for LTC are by those 80 years of age and older, with

Figure 27.1   Percent of United States Population 65 and Over,
1980–2030

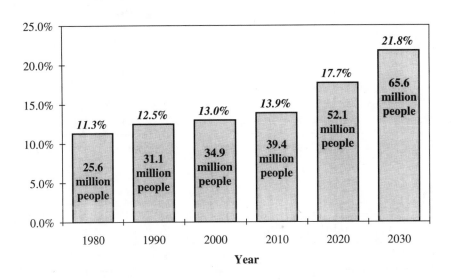

Source: C. M. Taeuber, *Sixty-Five Plus in America*, U.S. Department of Commerce, Bureau of the Census (Washington, DC) 1992.

55 percent of those 85 and above requiring at least one LTC service. More than half of the aged who live at home and require LTC receive no assistance. As shown in Figure 27.2, of those elderly men receiving assistance, the most frequent caregivers are family members, particularly the wife (37 percent); children (24 percent), usually daughters; other relatives (23 percent); and paid caregivers (16 percent). Women more often than men provide the uncompensated care. When the impaired aged is a woman, typically a widow, the most frequent caregivers are children and relatives. These services by family members, while uncompensated, are costly to the caregivers in terms of added strain on spouses and the need for their daughters to reduce their hours at work or leave their job.

The need for nursing home care also increases with age; 43 percent of the aged will use a nursing home at some point in their lives. At any point in time, approximately 5 percent of the aged (about 1.5 million) are in a nursing home. An estimated 1 percent of those aged 65–74 are in nursing homes, compared to 6 percent of those 75–84, and 22 percent of those 85 years and older (U.S. Senate Special Committee on

Table 27.1   Percent of the Aged Requiring Long-Term Care Services, 1987

Age Group	Percent
65 to 69	8.4
70 to 74	11.7
75 to 79	17.5
80 to 84	30.9
85 or older	54.8
65 or older	17.1

Source: U.S. Congressional Budget Office, *Policy Choices for Long-Term Care*, June 1991, Table 1, page 6.

Figure 27.2   Percent Distribution of Caregivers for People 65 Years and Older, 1982

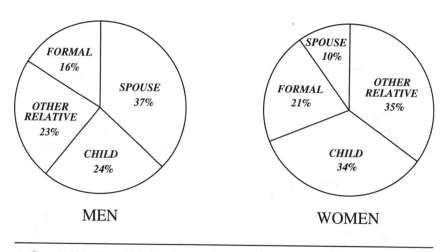

MEN   WOMEN

Source: U.S. Senate Special Committee on Aging, *Aging America: Trends and Projections, 1991 ed.*, p. 156.

Aging 1991, 162). The main reasons for nursing home use are severe functional deficiencies, mental disabilities (such as Alzheimer's), and lack of a family to provide services in the person's own home. The fastest-growing age group has been and will continue to be those over age 80, who will have the greatest needs for LTC and nursing homes.

The Current State of Long-Term Care Financing

The major sources of LTC financing are individuals and Medicaid programs. Currently, individuals and their families bear most of the burden for LTC out of their own resources, either out-of-pocket or as informal, unpaid caregivers. Medicare protects the aged from acute medical expenses but not from expenses incurred for chronic disability. Private LTC insurance is just beginning to increase, but presently only about 5 percent of the aged have such insurance. Medicaid pays for nursing home care and a limited amount of in-home coverage, but only after the impaired aged have exhausted their own financial resources. An individual is allowed to keep only $2,000. Current law permits a spouse to retain one-half of the couple's assets, up to a maximum of $70,000, inflation adjusted; including a private home of any value, if it is the principal residence.

To limit their Medicaid expenditures, states have limited the availability of nursing home beds, paid nursing homes low rates, and provided very limited in-home services to those eligible for Medicaid. The consequence of these policies has been a continual excess demand for nursing home beds by the impaired aged and low quality of services. Since few states pay nursing homes according to the level of care needed by the patient, nursing homes have an incentive to admit those Medicaid patients who have lower care needs and who are less costly to care for. And when a private-pay patient seeks nursing home care, they will be admitted before the Medicaid patient because their payment exceeds Medicaid reimbursement. As the demand by private patients increases, the excess demand by Medicaid patients will become larger.

The largest component of LTC services is for nursing homes, which represent 75 percent of LTC expenditures and have been increasing at 12.6 percent per year. The aged and their families pay, on average, 50 percent of all nursing home care (see Table 27.2).

Most of the aged who enter a nursing home will do so for a short period (see Table 27.3). But 18 percent of those who enter a nursing home will stay more than 2 years, in which case the financial burden is very large, exceeding $100,000. These 18 percent of the aged incur 89 percent of all nursing home costs. When a large number of people are at risk, but only few will incur a LTC catastrophic expense, insurance is a solution for those who can afford it.

The aged's fear of a nursing home stay that will deplete their lifetime savings and impoverish their spouse is one of the aged's major

Table 27.2   Estimated Spending on Long-Term Care Services by Type
of Service and Payment Source, 1988

Payment Source	Nursing Home Care	Home- and Community- Based Care	Total
	Billions of Dollars		
Total	44.3	13.6	57.8
Federal	13.3	5.0	18.3
Medicare	0.9	2.4	3.3
Medicaid	11.5	1.3	12.9
State and Local	9.5	2.6	12.1
Medicaid	9.4	1.1	10.5
Private	21.5	6.0	27.5
Out-of-Pocket	20.2	5.1	25.3
	Percent of Total		
Total	76.6%	23.5%	100.0%
Federal	30.0	36.8	31.7
Medicare	2.0	17.6	5.7
Medicaid	26.0	9.6	22.3
State and Local	21.4	19.1	20.9
Medicaid	21.2	8.1	18.2
Private	48.5	44.1	47.6
Out-of-Pocket	45.6	37.5	43.8

Source: U.S. Congressional Budget Office, *Policy Choices for Long-Term Care*, June
1991, Summary Table 1, p. xi.

reasons for desiring a federal LTC program. The middle-class aged would
like to bequeath their assets to their children rather than spend those assets
down to qualify for Medicaid. Low-income aged find it difficult to find a
nursing home willing to admit them. Further, if the aged have to go to a
nursing home, they would like it to be of high quality. The aged would
also rather be cared for in their own home than in a nursing home, but
are fearful of becoming a burden on their children. For the aged to be
provided with a range of LTC services, from in-home services to nursing
home care, without financially burdening them or their children, would
require huge government subsidies.

Table 27.3 Distribution of Expected Discounted Lifetime Nursing Home Cost

Lifetime Use	Percent of Cohort	Percent of Cost*
None	56.8	0.0
<3 months	11.4	1.0
3–6 months	3.6	1.1
6 months–1 year	4.8	2.8
1–2 years	5.2	6.5
2–5 years	9.4	24.7
5+ years	8.9	63.9
Total	100.0	100.0

*Percentage of cost incurred by persons in each category of lifetime use.
Reprinted with permission, as it appeared in P. Kemper, B. C. Spillman, and C. M. Murtaugh, "A Lifetime Perspective on Proposals for Financing Nursing Home Care," *Inquiry* 28 (Winter): 338. © 1991, the Blue Cross and Blue Shield Association.

The amount spent on nursing homes is about 1 percent of this country's gross domestic product output. Given the rapid increase in both the number and proportion of aged, federal subsidies to all the aged for their nursing home care and in-home services will be a very large burden on the non-aged.

What should be the role of government in financing LTC for the aged? Should all aged be subsidized, or should subsidies be targeted to low-income aged? And who should bear the burden of taxes for the level of government expenditures that would be required to fund these different-sized government programs?

Private Sector Approach

A private sector approach would place primary responsibility on the individual and the family. The government would fill the gap between the elderly's needs and what their family and financial resources can provide. Availability of government assistance would be based, as Medicaid does, on the elderly's income and assets. The government would inform the aged about their needs for LTC insurance and the lack of such coverage in Medicare and "Medigap" policies (which cover the deductibles and copayments included in Medicare). Currently, about 70 percent of the aged purchase "Medigap" policies, which cost about $70 a month; LTC insurance would cost about $100 a month (for ages 65–74), which 50 percent of the aged are estimated to be able to afford.

Social Insurance Approach

"Social insurance" advocates believe the financial burden and the anxiety placed on family and friends is too great not to be shared by society. These advocates would require everyone to contribute (through taxes) to fund an LTC program, which would then be available to all aged, regardless of economic status, when they need it (for further readings in this area, see Cohen et al. 1992; Scanlon 1992; Wiener and Hanley 1991; Congressional Budget Office 1991).

Back-end Coverage

Two types of social insurance approaches for meeting the aged's LTC needs have been proposed. The "back end" coverage approach would provide government subsidies for nursing home care (without requiring a Medicaid spend-down requirement) after the person has paid the first two years of care themselves. This is the same as a government insurance policy with a large deductible. As shown in Table 27.3, 89 percent of nursing home costs are incurred by 18 percent of the aged, who stay longer than two years. Back-end coverage would commit the government to pick up 89 percent of all nursing home expenses, regardless of the aged's wealth. The estimated cost of this subsidy would be $35 billion (based on the government paying only 80 percent of nursing home and home care costs after a two-year deductible). The main beneficiaries of a back-end policy would be the wealthier aged who would no longer need to purchase private LTC insurance to protect their assets.

Front-end Coverage

The second approach, "front end" coverage, would cover the first year of nursing home care for all the aged, regardless of the aged's income or assets; this approach is similar to first-dollar insurance coverage. The estimated subsidy required to fund this program would be $39 billion, which also assumes lifetime home care benefits (Cohen et al. 1992). Even though the financial burden of a long stay is very large for the individual, because many aged would have short nursing home stays, a front-end subsidy is very expensive. While low-income aged would benefit, most of the subsidy would again accrue to those with higher incomes. Covering all the aged, regardless of income or wealth, increases the cost of such a program. Relatively short stays in the nursing home are more affordable to most of the aged than long stays, which are likely to impoverish most of the aged. Under front-end coverage the aged would still be at risk for catastrophic nursing home expenses.

Redistributive Effects

Each of these approaches for subsidizing the aged's LTC expenses have redistributive effects, in that some income groups will be taxed to provide benefits to other income groups. One must determine whether these redistributive effects improve or worsen equity. For example, should all taxpayers (possibly through a sales tax), many of whom would have low and middle incomes, subsidize the nursing home costs of middle- and high-income aged to enable them to leave their assets to their children? Unless government subsidies are targeted to those aged with the lowest incomes and assets, such subsidies are likely to be inequitable and should be viewed more as asset protection programs for the middle class.

Other Effects

In addition to equity effects, these public subsidies will affect the demand for private LTC insurance. If the aged are no longer responsible for a major portion of their LTC expenses, the aged will be less likely to purchase LTC insurance. A more-appropriate public policy might be to encourage the purchase of private LTC insurance by those who can afford to do so and to use limited public funds for others.

If Medicare and Medicaid history is any guide, as the cost of the program increases, a government-funded LTC program will eventually limit payments to nursing homes and access to in-home services. Unless government nursing home payments are adequate, there will be an insufficient supply to serve the growing number of aged. The government will be reluctant to include generous in-home services ($50 to $200 a day) as part of an LTC policy because home care is unlikely to merely substitute for costly nursing home stays but would, instead, increase total LTC expenses.

Whenever the price of a service is reduced, as through a subsidy, the use of that service will increase. More impaired aged would enter nursing homes rather than remain on their own and paid caregivers will substitute for informal caregivers. An evaluation of a government-funded LTC program to all aged should consider whether the tax requirements of such a program will cause the government to eventually limit access to care, as has occurred with Medicaid.

Mixed Approaches

Refundable Tax Credits

There are two mixed government and private approaches that might also be considered. A refundable tax credit (which declines as incomes increase) to those who purchase LTC insurance targets the low-income aged and would alleviate the concern that the government would reduce the aged's access in order to limit its expenditures. It is refundable in the sense that if the person's tax liability is less than the tax credit, the person receives a refund once he or she provides proof of purchase of an approved LTC insurance policy. Those with higher incomes who can afford to purchase LTC insurance would not receive a subsidy. The benefits of the tax subsidy would go to those with lower incomes and would stimulate the purchase of LTC insurance.

Medical Individual Retirement Accounts

Similar to the above would be to allow individuals to deduct from their adjusted gross income contributions (up to $2,000 per year) to a "medical individual retirement account" (MIRA), which could be used upon retirement for LTC expenses, as well as for other retirement needs. Making contributions to MIRAs tax-exempt are an incentive for individuals to make such contributions. The eventual size of these investments would, at retirement, alleviate the aged's concern with their LTC expenses. If a government subsidy is provided to those unable to make such contributions, then the cost of the program would consist of such subsidies as well as the loss in tax revenues from such deductions from adjusted gross income. This program would be more costly than a refundable tax credit discussed above. Again, to limit the loss of tax revenues, the amount of the contribution that is tax-exempt should, as with the tax credit, decline the higher the person's income.

Private Long-Term Care Insurance

Dependence on Medicaid and the need for government LTC subsidies would diminish if more of the aged purchased private LTC insurance. Yet less than 5 percent of the aged have LTC insurance. Why hasn't private LTC insurance grown more rapidly? And how feasible is it to expect private LTC insurance to alleviate the middle-class aged's concerns with LTC?

When individuals are subject to large unexpected expenses, there is a demand for insurance. A private insurance market then develops that enables individuals to reduce their financial risk in exchange for a premium. Given the growing number of aged at risk for financially catastrophic nursing home (and in-home) costs, the potential market for LTC insurance is huge. There are, however, several reasons why such a small percent of the aged have bought LTC insurance.

First, there is a great deal of misinformation among the aged—many believe Medicare and "Medigap" insurance also cover LTC services (they do not). Second, the aged's income and ability to pay for LTC insurance are quite variable. The oldest old, those most in need of LTC, generally have lower incomes than the younger aged and are in a higher-risk group; consequently, their insurance premiums are much higher. If the older aged need to enter a nursing home, they have to rely on Medicaid, which is their low-cost LTC insurance.

Another important reason for the low demand for private LTC insurance is the relatively high loading charge that is added to the premium. The higher the loading charge, relative to the pure premium (expected claims experience), the lower the demand for such insurance. The marketing and administrative costs of selling LTC insurance to individuals is much higher than if such insurance were sold to large employer groups.

Also increasing the loading charge is insurers' concern with adverse selection. LTC insurance is sold to individuals on a voluntary basis, whereas employer-paid health insurance includes everyone in the group, which eliminates the chance that only sick employees will buy the insurance. Since insurance premiums are based on the average expected claims experience (use rate multiplied by the price of the service) of a particular age/sex group, insurers are concerned that a higher proportion of the impaired aged will buy the LTC insurance. It is costly for insurers to examine each potential purchaser of LTC insurance to determine whether he or she has impairments that will require assistance. This "testing," if it were performed, would further increase the loading charge relative to the pure premium, thereby decreasing the demand for such insurance by lower-risk subscribers. Instead, "delay of benefits" provisions are included to discourage adverse selection.

Insurers are also concerned that as insurance becomes available to pay for in-home services, the demand for such services will sharply increase. Ideally, LTC insurance should provide comprehensive services, both in-home assistance as well as nursing home care. It would be less expensive to provide in-home services (as well as being preferred by the impaired aged) when it reduces use of the more-expensive nursing home. Currently, many of the impaired aged do not receive any assistance from others. The aged's use of services to meet this unmet need will increase as insurance becomes available to pay for in-home services. Further, those impaired aged that receive in-home services are generally assisted by family members without charge. Once insurance becomes available, paid caregivers might substitute for family members. It is uncertain how large this shift might be, but, unless controlled, it could have a large effect on the insurer's cost, and consequently on the premium.

To protect themselves from the claims experience that could result from comprehensive LTC coverage, insurers have imposed a six-month preexisting condition clause and have required the aged to bear a portion of their LTC costs. Typically, an LTC policy will provide indemnity coverage of $40 a day for home health care and $80 a day for care in a nursing home, after the patient has met a "deductible" of 20 days in the nursing home. Many insurers limit nursing home coverage to four years.

Ideally, insurers (and the government as part of its LTC programs) should employ case managers to evaluate the aged's needs and determine the mix of services to be provided. In-home services could then be substituted for more-expensive nursing home care, and the discretionary use of the in-home assistance can be minimized. Until the problems of adverse selection and the discretionary aspects of in-home services can be solved, LTC insurance is likely to emphasize indemnity coverage, include a large deductible, and have a "delay of benefits" period before the coverage becomes effective.

Since the late 1980s, insurers have begun marketing LTC insurance to large employee groups. Group policies have lower loading charges because of their lower administrative and marketing costs. Adverse selection is also less of a concern when everyone in a group participates, particularly when they are at low risk for LTC. Further, since employees would not be at risk for many years, group LTC policies could be sold at very low premiums. Employer-sponsored LTC policies may be a useful financing source for future rather than current aged. However, unless older employees are better informed about their LTC risks and the costs of meeting those needs, they may not buy employer-sponsored LTC insurance when it is sold at low premiums.

Life-Care Communities

"Life-care communities," which combine LTC insurance and living facilities, are another alternative available to middle- and high-income aged. In return for a large entrance fee and a monthly payment, an aged individual or couple are promised care for the rest of their lives in a life-care community. They live independently in a home or apartment, and when their needs require it, they receive in-home assistance. A quality nursing home is also available when needed.

Summary

It has been estimated that less than 40 percent of the aged will be able to afford private LTC insurance. While this percentage indicates how large the private insurance market can become, it also indicates that there will be a sizable number unable to purchase insurance or other LTC services such as life-care communities.

LTC policy requires choices to be made. The aged have greater needs for care, do not wish to be a burden on family members, and do not want to spend down their hard-earned assets. Yet, given the projected number of aged, government LTC subsidies can be very costly, they will require large tax increases (particularly when the number of workers per aged person is declining, from 3.3 employees per aged today to 2.8 in 20 years), and they cause inequities between those benefiting and those bearing the cost of the social program. Subsidies also reduce the incentive for many aged to rely on their children and to purchase private LTC insurance. To reduce the cost of LTC subsidies, they should be targeted to those with low incomes, and workers and the aged should be educated about the need to protect themselves against catastrophic LTC costs.

References

Cohen, M. A., N. Kumar, T. McGuire, and S. Wallack. "Financing Long Term Care: A Practical Mix of Public and Private." *Journal of Health Politics, Policy and Law* 17 (Fall 1992): 403–23.

Scanlon, W. J. "Possible Reforms for Financing Long-Term Care." *The Journal of Economic Perspectives* 6 (Summer 1992): 43–58.

Wiener, J. M., and R. J. Hanley. "Long Term Care Financing: Problems and Progress." *Annual Review of Public Health* 12 (1991): 67–84.

U.S. Congress. Senate Special Committee on Aging. *Aging America: Trends and Projections.* Washington, DC: U.S. Government Printing Office, 1991.

U.S. Congressional Budget Office, *Policy Choices for Long-Term Care.* Washington, DC: Congressional Budget Office, 1991.

28

The Politics of Health Care Reform

There is great dissatisfaction with this country's health care system. More than 35 million do not have health insurance, hospitals and physicians are inadequately reimbursed for providing care to the poor, many fear losing their health insurance if they become ill, and the insured find themselves forced to join health plans that restrict their use of physicians, although they are paying higher premiums and more out-of-pocket for their medical care. Despite these constraints, the rapid rise of medical expenditures continues.

Health care has achieved high visibility in the media. Opinion polls indicate that the public wants national health insurance, health care reform was a prominent issue in the recent presidential election, and President Clinton placed health care reform high on his domestic agenda. Given public dissatisfaction with the current health system and apparent political support for those politicians who favor its reform, why is it so difficult to achieve national health insurance?

Advocates for health care reform want to receive benefits in excess of their costs, and the only way they can achieve this is if the government legislates it. However, if most groups are to have net benefits, some group will be stuck with paying the costs of those benefits. Which group in society will bear the added costs or taxes? Whichever group has to pay more will oppose legislators who vote to raise their taxes. The major difficulty in health care reform is finding groups that can be taxed to provide net benefits to politically powerful constituencies.

In the past, politically important groups received visible redistributive benefits that less politically powerful groups were taxed to provide.

To lessen the opposition of those being taxed, the tax was hidden. For example, splitting the Social Security tax between the employer and the employee makes it appear that the employee bears only one-half of the tax. In reality, economists believe most of the employer share is shifted back to the employee in the form of lower wages and that the rest is shifted forward to consumers as higher prices for goods and services.

To understand the difficulties of health care reform and what compromises are likely to emerge, one must examine the goals of different political constituencies. In doing so, it soon becomes obvious that national health insurance means different things to different groups.

The Differing Goals of Health Care Reform

Many assume the main purpose of national health insurance is to increase the availability of medical services to those with low incomes.

Certainly many individuals support increased services to the poor, but this is not, nor has it ever been, the driving force behind NHI— Medicaid is NHI for the poor. To use the power of government to achieve one's objectives requires political power. The inadequate structure and funding of Medicaid is indicative of the limited political power of the poor and their advocates. These inadequacies are not due to the actions of a few miserly bureaucrats or legislators but are, instead, reflective of the resources that society—the middle class—is willing to devote to the poor. States vary in their generosity and in criteria used for determining Medicaid eligibility. No state reaches the federal poverty level in determining Medicaid eligibility, and some states are at only 25 percent of it. How much the nonpoor will spend on charity depends on how much the nonpoor themselves have, on how culturally similar the poor are to the nonpoor, and on how much it costs to provide for the poor.

Since it is the nonpoor who have the political power to determine the allocation of resources to the poor, one must assume that the inadequacies of Medicaid are reflections of insufficient interest among the nonpoor in improving Medicaid and increasing funding for the poor. If society is unwilling to improve Medicaid, why would they tax themselves to enact NHI for the poor?

If, then, NHI is not primarily for the poor, its broader purpose must be to use the power of government to benefit politically powerful groups. Politically influential groups have a "concentrated" interest in a particular issue and are able to organize themselves to provide political support to legislators, that is, campaign contributions, votes, and volunteer time. A group is said to have a concentrated interest if specific regulation or legislation potentially will affect that group enough to make it worthwhile for the group to invest resources either to forestall or to promote that effect. The potential legislative benefits must exceed the group's costs of organizing and providing political support.

Implicit in this discussion of concentrated interests is the assumption that legislators will respond to political support since their objective is to be reelected. It is assumed that legislators are similar to the other participants in the policy process and that, rationally, they undertake cost-benefit calculations of their actions. However, they weigh the political support gained and lost by their legislative actions, not the legislation's effect on society.

Initially, physicians and hospitals were the major groups in the health field with a concentrated interest in health legislation. Payment systems under both public and private insurance systems had a large effect on their revenues, and competitors (such as HMOs, PPOs, outpatient surgery centers, foreign-trained physicians) also affected hospital and physician revenues. These financial concerns, related to demand for services, methods of pricing, the availability of substitutes to their services, and their overall supply, prompted physician and hospital associations to represent (successfully) their concentrated interests before both state and federal legislatures. One demonstration of the American Medical Association's (AMA) political power was the defeat of President Truman's proposed NHI plan. Legislators who had opposed the AMA's economic interests found the AMA a force to be reckoned with at election time.

These legislative actions by physician and hospital associations were neither very obvious nor, initially, very costly to the consumers of medical services. While medical prices rose faster than they would have otherwise, alternatives to the fee-for-service system, such as managed care, were unavailable. These costs to consumers were not sufficiently large to make it worthwhile for them to organize, represent their interests before legislatures, and offer political support to those legislators favorable to their interests.

The concentrated interests of medical providers and the subsequent diffuse (small) costs imposed on consumers explain much of the legislative history on the financing and delivery of medical services until the early 1960s.

The enactment and design of Medicare illustrates the real purpose of NHI: to redistribute wealth, that is, to increase benefits to politically powerful groups, without their paying the full costs of those benefits, by shifting the costs to the less politically powerful.

Throughout the 1950s and early 1960s, the AFL-CIO unions had a concentrated interest in their retirees' medical costs that placed them in opposition to the AMA. Employers had not prefunded union retirees' medical costs, but paid them instead as part of current labor expenses. If union retirees' medical expenses could be shifted away from the employer, then those same funds would be available to be paid as higher wages to union employees. To ensure that their union retirees would be eligible for Medicare, the unions insisted Medicare (hospital services) be financed via Social Security, and it was this attempt to shift costs onto others that became the central issue in the debate over Medicare (see Feldstein 1988). The AMA was willing to have government assistance go only to those unable to afford medical services, which would have increased the demand for physicians. Thus, the AMA favored a means-tested program funded by general tax revenues because it was concerned that subsidies to the nonpoor would merely substitute government payment for private payment. Such a program would cost too much, leading to controls on hospital and physician fees.

With the landslide victory of President Johnson in 1964, the unions achieved their objective. Once Social Security financing was used to determine eligibility for Medicare, Medicare Part B (physician services) was added, financed by general tax revenues.

Although the unions won on the financing mechanism, the Congress acceded to the demands of the medical and hospital associations on all other aspects of the legislation. The system of payment to hospitals and physicians promoted inefficiency (cost-plus payments to hospitals), and restrictions limiting competition were placed on alternative delivery systems. This historic conflict between opposing concentrated interests in medical care left both victorious and depicts how the power of government can be used to benefit politically important groups. As a result of Medicare, a massive redistribution of wealth occurred in society. The beneficiaries were the aged, union members, and medical providers, financed by a diffuse tax (Social Security) over a large group, the working population, who also paid higher prices for their medical services and more income taxes to finance Medicare Part B.

Medicare was designed to be both inefficient and inequitable, simply because it was in the economic interests of those with concentrated interests.

Groups Having a Concentrated Interest in Change

Today, many more groups have a concentrated interest in health legislation. To understand the conflicting forces pressuring for change and NHI, however, one has to examine the objectives of several of the more important groups.

Federal and State Governments

Since Medicare and Medicaid were enacted in 1965, every administration has been confronted with rapidly rising Medicare and Medicaid expenditures. As expenditures greatly exceeded projections, what had initially been a diffuse cost became a concentrated cost to successive administrations. Each administration faced choices with potentially high political costs. To prevent the Medicare Trust Fund from going bankrupt, the administration could reduce benefits to the aged, increase Social Security taxes, or pay hospitals less. No choice was without political costs, but increasing Social Security taxes and placing limits on how much hospitals were to be paid was considered less costly than reducing benefits to the aged.

To continue funding rapidly rising Medicaid expenditures, which are funded from general tax revenues, the states chose to limit Medicaid eligibility and to reduce their payments to health providers rather than to reduce other politically popular programs or to increase taxes. However, the percent of the poor served by Medicaid declined, as did the participation of physicians and hospitals.

Medicare Part B, funded by general tax revenues, contributes to the federal budget deficit. As these expenditures have risen, each administration's choices have been limited. Increasing taxes and creating a larger deficit are both politically costly, as is increasing the aged's contribution (they currently pay 25 percent of the premium); the only other alternative was to pay physicians less and to place them (as of 1993) under a volume-expenditure limit.

Federal and state administrations have developed a concentrated interest in holding down the rise in government expenditures, which has placed them in conflict with hospital and physician organizations. Currently, government health policies appear to be concerned primarily with limiting Medicare and Medicaid expenditures. Politically, the least costly approach is to pay providers less. Only under Medicaid are the politically weak beneficiaries also adversely affected.

Employers and Unions

Rising employee medical expenses became a concern to employers and their unions in the 1980s because of more-intense import competition. No longer could these companies merely increase their prices to compensate for higher employee health costs as they had previously done; there would have been large reductions in sales and, consequently, in union employees. Although union membership has fallen from 25 percent of the workforce in 1972 to 14.5 percent in 1990, unions have greater political influence than their numbers suggest; they are organized and are able to offer large contributions to attain their economic interests. A lower rate of increase in health costs would permit their union members to receive greater wage increases. Thus unions have favored proposals to limit medical expenditure increases.

Similarly, a recent ruling by the Financial Accounting Standards Board (FASB) has stimulated several corporations, such as Chrysler, to promote NHI. The FASB ruling requires employers who provide their retirees with medical benefits to add that liability to their balance sheet starting in 1993. This liability would have to include the full estimate of their retirees' future medical expenses and the estimated retiree benefit liability for their current employees, as well. Currently, retiree medical benefits are an unfunded liability to those large corporations that provide such benefits. The employer pays retiree medical costs as they occur, treating them as current expenses. Placing this entire liability on the balance sheet reduces the net worth of many major corporations by a significant amount. Their equity per share will drop substantially. In addition, corporate earnings will decline, since a portion of this retiree liability for medical benefits (both for retirees and for current employees) will have to be expensed annually.

Any NHI plan that restricts the growth of medical expenditures will limit the size of corporations' unfunded retiree medical liabilities (particularly the automobile companies) and permit larger increases in employee wages.

Physicians and Hospitals

The influence of physician and hospital associations has declined as other groups (particularly the federal and state governments) have developed a concentrated interest in limiting medical expenditures. The objective of hospitals and physicians, as opposed to that of the federal and state governments and employers, is to have increased medical expenditures. Today, the strongest lobbyists for financing medical care to the poor are hospitals, since they stand to gain additional revenues.

The Aged

The aged have NHI for acute care (Medicare), but their most pressing concern (for the middle- and high-income aged) is for protection from the costs of long-term care. An extended stay in a nursing home depletes the assets of many of the aged. Medicare covers neither long-term care nor nursing home care unrelated to acute illness. The aged with low incomes must rely on Medicaid for long-term care. An aged person whose assets exceed the Medicaid limit must "spend down" those assets to qualify for Medicaid. Government-subsidized long-term care insurance would protect the assets of the aged. Rather than purchasing such asset protection in the marketplace, the aged prefer government legislation that would shift part of their costs to other population groups. The aged, who have high voting participation rates, thereby increasing their political influence, also have the support of the near aged (who would soon benefit from new aged benefits) as well as of their children.

The repeal of the Medicare Catastrophic Act illustrates the true purpose of redistributive legislation. In 1988 Congress thought the aged would be appreciative of their efforts to provide them with protection against catastrophic acute care while financing this new benefit by charging a higher Part B premium to the higher-income aged. However, the high-income aged had already purchased such protection privately ("Medigap" insurance) and did not want to pay higher premiums just to support lower-income aged. The middle- and high-income aged vigorously protested this increased tax until the act was repealed the next year.

The Middle Class

The middle class (those in the middle-income group) have a disproportionately large amount of political power since they are the median voters. It is difficult to form a majority of voters without those in the middle. If national health insurance were a highly visible issue, around which there was consensus, and it was strongly supported by the middle class, legislators would respond to the potential political support that would be forthcoming. It is instructive, therefore, to consider why the middle class has not been a strong supporter of NHI.

Rapidly rising medical costs have, until recently, been a diffuse cost to the middle class. Tax-free employer-paid health insurance has insulated employees and their families from the rising costs of medical care. For example, an increase of $1,000 in income is worth more to the employee if it is not first reduced by federal, state, and Social Security taxes. High rates of inflation pushed employees into high marginal tax brackets during the 1970s, providing them with an incentive to increase their insurance coverage rather than paying dental, vision, and other medical expenses out-of-pocket with after-tax dollars. Until the last several years, employees have had unlimited choice of providers, limited cost-sharing, and small, if any, copremiums. According to a 1989 survey conducted by the Bureau of Labor Statistics, 53 percent of medium and large employers still pay the full health insurance premium for their employees, and 34 percent for families.

Tax-free employer-paid health insurance has been a form of NHI for middle- and high-income groups. The forgone tax revenue of employer-paid health insurance premiums is currently estimated to be $60 billion. Given the significant tax advantages of employer-paid premiums and the fact that increased employer-paid premiums have not visibly lowered their wages, middle- and high-income employees have been insulated from rising medical costs; NHI has therefore not been an important financial issue. Employees have probably been at greater financial risk for the long-term care needs of their aged parents than for their own acute care needs.

Polls have come up with some surprising and seemingly contradictory findings on American attitudes toward a "national health plan." For example, 89 percent of the Americans surveyed see the need for fundamental reform of the U.S. health care system, yet employees and their families are satisfied with the care they receive from their physicians and hospitals. They are not concerned with how much is spent on health care in the United States, and employees enjoy their free choice of physicians and hospitals. What can one conclude from these surveys? The public was not asked to make any trade-offs. They were led to believe they could have the best of the current system at a lower cost. When they were asked whether they were willing to pay more, their support for a comprehensive national health system declined.

Dissatisfaction with our current system is, however, increasing as the middle class pays higher out-of-pocket payments and are forced into more-restrictive health plans. Basically, the public would like to pay less for their health care and not be concerned about losing their health insurance if they lose or change jobs.

The conflicting objectives of the above groups explains the lack of consensus about what NHI should achieve. Federal and state governments, large employers, and unions want to limit medical expenditure increases. The once politically powerful physician and hospital associations want increased medical expenditures. The aged, who have national health insurance for acute care, want a new long-term care program whose costs would be borne by others. The middle class want what they have now, at least, but at a lower cost.

The Likely Structure and Financing of National Health Insurance

As medical expenditures continue to rise, employers are shifting a greater portion of their health insurance premiums to employees and requiring larger deductibles and cost-sharing in their insurance plans. Employers are also choosing more-restrictive health plans, such as HMOs, PPOs, and EPOs (exclusive provider organizations), to limit medical expenditure increases. As this continues, legislators have recognized that NHI has become a visible political issue worthy of middle-class political support. To be politically salable to the middle class, any NHI proposal must promise them benefits in excess of their costs; that is, they will pay less but receive the same medical services.

It is for these reasons that the Clinton administration has based its NHI proposal around two important concepts. The first is mandating employers to provide their employees with health insurance. Most employees without health insurance earn low wages and work in small firms having fewer than 25 employees; small employers are the main opposition to this legislation. The federal and state governments favor this approach since it would shift medical costs off the Medicaid budget. Hospital and physician associations also favor this approach since it would increase the demand for their services. Many large employers and their unions also support mandating employer coverage because it would increase the labor costs of low-cost competitors, while not placing any additional burdens on their own employees' medical costs. The middle class is unlikely to oppose an employer mandate since it would not explicitly increase their taxes and appears to be a means of providing health insurance to low-wage employees by shifting their costs onto employers. In actuality, the burden would fall mostly on low-wage employees.

Mandated employer health insurance, while politically feasible, is not, however, NHI. It does nothing to limit the increase in medical expenditures, which is a major objective of the federal and state governments, unions, and large employers. More importantly, an employer mandate would provide no visible net benefits to the middle class nor would it reduce their rising premiums and out-of-pocket expenses, which would be the basis of their support for NHI. Thus, under the Clinton administration proposal an employer mandate is combined with an artificial limit on the rise in insurance and HMO premiums, which would limit the growth in hospital, physician, and total health care expenditures. Under such expenditure limits, the middle class are promised that they would receive all the services they now receive and at lower prices. They would not be required to make any sacrifices. The resources to provide all the necessary services would come from reduced "waste" in the current system.

Expenditure caps on providers also serve the interests of unions, employers, and the federal and state governments (who are already using this approach). The main opposition to this approach has been from physicians and hospitals, who would receive less revenues.

Combining an employer mandate with expenditure limits on physicians, hospitals, and HMOs is politically attractive as long as the public can be misled into believing that they can have greater access to care at no additional cost by merely reducing waste. The uninsured would be provided insurance by requiring their employer to pay the premium. It would not be obvious to the middle class that low-wage employees would, in fact, be taxed to bear most of the burden of their own insurance. Large employers and unions would benefit, as would the federal and state governments, as a portion of their Medicaid costs would be shifted onto small employers and their employees.

The structure and financing of national health insurance becomes a consequence of the economic interests of politically powerful groups. To forecast the likely financing and structure of the delivery system, it is not as important to understand which methods of taxation are more equitable, what their effects are on employment, or which delivery systems are more efficient, as it is to understand the political feasibility of different alternatives.

NHI could be achieved by using a price-competitive market in which managed care plans compete for subscribers. Those with low incomes would be given income-related vouchers for use in a managed care plan. The rise in health care expenditures would be determined by market competition. However, a market approach has not been proposed by the administration because it does not provide visible benefits to the middle class. Further, to provide the poor with subsidies to join managed care plans would require the government to pay the market price charged by such plans, necessitating increased taxes.

As long the public is led to believe that it is possible for them to have all the care they want without paying for it, equitable and efficient health care reform is unlikely to occur. The problem with coming to grips with serious reform is not with special interest groups, but with the middle class; they need to recognize that it is necessary to make a trade-off between access to services and the amount they are willing to pay.

Reference

Feldstein, P. J. *The Politics of Health Legislation: An Economic Perspective.* Ann Arbor, MI: Health Administration Press, 1988. (See Chapter 9, "Medicare.")

Appendix: Discussion Questions

Chapter 1. The Rise in Medical Expenditures

1. What are some of the reasons for the increase in demand for medical services since 1965?

2. Why has employer-paid health insurance been an important stimulant of demand for health insurance?

3. How did hospital payment methods in the 1960s and 1970s affect hospitals' incentives for efficiency and investment policy?

4. Why weren't HMOs and managed care more prevalent in the 1960s and 1970s?

5. What were the federal government's choices to reduce the greater-than-projected Medicare expenditures?

6. What events occurred during the 1980s in both the public and private sectors to make the delivery of medical services price competitive?

Chapter 2. How Much Should We Spend on Medical Care?

1. How does a competitive market determine the types of goods and services to be produced, how much it costs to produce those goods, and who receives them?

2. Why do economists believe that the value of additional employer-paid health insurance is worth less than its full cost?

3. Why is there concern over the rise in medical expenditures?

4. What are the reasons for inefficiencies in the demand and provision of medical services?

5. Why are large employers and government concerned over rising medical expenditures?

Chapter 3. Do More Medical Expenditures Produce Better Health?

1. How can a health production function be used for allocating funds to improve health levels?

2. Why does this country spend an increasing portion of its resources on medical services even though it is less cost-effective than other methods for improving health levels?

3. How can employers use the concept of a health production function for decreasing their employees' medical expenditures?

4. Describe a production function for decreasing deaths from coronary heart disease.

5. Describe a production function for decreasing deaths of young adults.

Chapter 4. In Whose Interest Does the Physician Act?

1. Why do physicians play such a crucial role in the delivery of medical services?

2. How might a decrease in physician incomes, possibly as a result of an increase in the number of physicians, affect their role as the patient's agent?

3. What are some of the ways in which insurers seek to compensate for the information advantage that physicians have?

4. What forces currently serve to limit "supplier-induced demand"?

5. How do fee-for-service and capitation payment systems affect the physician's role as the patient's agent?

Chapter 5. Rationing Medical Services

1. What determines how many physician services an individual would demand?

2. What is "moral hazard," and how does its existence increase the cost of medical care?

3. What are the various ways that moral hazard can be limited?

4. If medical services were free but the government restricted the supply of services so that physician office visits were rationed by waiting time, what population groups would fare better?

5. How would you use information on price sensitivity of medical services for policy purposes, for example, to increase the use of mammograms?

6. Discuss: The high price sensitivity of health plan copremiums indicates that if employees had to pay out-of-pocket the difference between the lowest-cost health plan and any other health plan, market competition among health plans would be stimulated.

Chapter 6. How Much Health Insurance Should Everyone Have?

1. How is a "pure premium" calculated?

2. What does the loading charge consist of?

3. How does the size of the loading charge affect the type of health insurance purchased?

4. Why does employer-purchased health insurance result in more-comprehensive health insurance coverage?

5. What are the arguments in favor of eliminating the tax-exempt status of employer-purchased health insurance?

6. How has health insurance affected the development of medical technology, and how has medical technology affected the growth of health insurance?

Chapter 7. Why Are Those Who Most Need Health Insurance Least Able to Buy It?

1. What are the different components of a health insurance premium? If an employer wanted to reduce their employees' premiums, which components could be changed?

2. What is "adverse selection," and how do insurance companies protect themselves from it? What would be the effect on insurance premiums if the government prohibited insurers from protecting themselves from adverse selection?

3. Why do insurers and HMOs have an incentive to engage in "preferred-risk selection"?

4. What are some methods by which insurers and HMOs try to achieve preferred-risk selection?

5. What is the difference between "experience" rating and "community" rating, and what are some consequences of using community rating?

Chapter 8. Medicare and Medicaid

1. What are the differences between Medicare and Medicaid?

2. How well does Medicaid achieve its objectives?

3. How equitable are the methods used to finance Medicare?

4. How does the Medicare Hospital Trust Fund differ from a pension fund?

5. How might the financing of Medicare be changed so that only low-income aged are subsidized?

Chapter 9. The New Medicare Physician Payment System

1. What were the reasons for developing a new Medicare physician payment system?

2. In what ways does the new physician payment system differ from the previous system?

3. What are likely to be the effects on Medicare patients' out-of-pocket expenses, Part B premiums, and access to physicians (primary care versus specialists) of the new payment system?

4. What, if any, are the likely effects on patients in the non-Medicare (private) sector?

5. What are the likely effects of the new payment system on physicians (by specialty)?

Chapter 10. Physician Incomes

1. Why did patients become less price sensitive to physician fee increases since the 1960s?

2. Why have the incomes of surgical specialists increased faster than those of primary care physicians?

3. What trends are occurring in the physician services market to suggest that the income trends of surgical specialists and primary care physicians will be different in the 1990s than they were in the 1980s?

4. Why has the size of multispecialty medical groups been increasing?

5. There are two basic reasons why prices change in a competitive market. In what way are these reasons applicable for explaining physician fee increases?

Chapter 11. The Malpractice Crisis

1. How well does the malpractice system compensate victims of negligence?

2. How effective is the deterrence function of the malpractice system?

3. Discuss the advantages and disadvantages of "no fault" insurance.

4. Do you think that the costs of "defensive medicine" would be reduced under a "no fault" system?

5. Evaluate the effects on deterrence and victim compensation of the following:

   a. Limits on lawyers' contingency fees

   b. Excluding testimony from out-of-state experts

   c. Limits on the size of malpractice awards

   d. Placing the liability for malpractice on the health care organization to which the physician belongs

Chapter 12. Competition among Hospitals: Does It Raise or Lower Costs?

1. Why did hospital expenditures rise so rapidly after the introduction of Medicare and Medicaid in 1966?

2. What changes did Medicare DRGs cause in hospital behavior?

3. What is the response of hospitals likely to be when the hospital is the only hospital in the market compared to when there are ten hospitals competing for a large employer's employees?

4. What determines the number of competitors in a market? Apply your answer to obstetrics and to transplant services.

5. What are some anticompetitive hospital actions that the antitrust laws seek to prevent?

Chapter 13. Vertically Integrated Health Care Organizations

1. Describe the changing costs and benefits of different organizational structures in the period before the 1980s.

2. What forces have been most important in causing the hospital to change its organizational structure?

3. What are "transactions costs" and how did they encourage hospitals to purchase nursing homes after the introduction of Medicare DRGs?

4. How did Medicare DRGs and capitation increase the interdependence between hospitals and physicians?

5. When a hospital becomes a cost center in a capitated organization rather than a revenue center under fee-for-service, how would the hospital administrator's behavior be expected to change?

Chapter 14. Cost Shifting

1. Explain why an increase in a hospital's fixed costs or an increase in the number of uninsured cared for by the hospital will not change the hospital's profit-maximizing price.

2. Why would a change in a hospital's variable costs change the hospital's profit-maximizing price?

3. Why are hospitals able to charge different purchasers different prices for the same medical services?

4. Under what circumstances can cost shifting occur?

5. How does cost shifting differ from price discrimination?

Chapter 15. Can Price Controls Limit Medical Expenditure Increases?

1. Why do price controls cause shortages, and why do these shortages increase over time?

2. Why do price controls require hospitals to make a trade-off between quality of medical services and number of patients served?

3. What are the various ways in which a provider can "game" the system under price controls?

4. What "costs" do price controls impose on patients?

5. What are the advantages and disadvantages of permitting patients to "buy out" of the price-controlled medical system?

Chapter 16. Managed Care Competition

1. Provide examples of the different types of managed care organizations and explain how they differ.

2. What is the difference between managed care competition and managed competition? What are the pros and cons of each form of competition?

3. Why do advocates of competition claim that it has not yet been tried in health care?

4. How would an advocate of managed care competition evaluate the Clinton administration's proposal for managed competition?

6. Why is a regulated health care system, such as exists in Canada and as proposed by the Clinton administration, able to achieve a lower rate of increase in medical expenditures than would occur under managed care competition?

Chapter 17. American Competitiveness and Rising Health Costs

1. What determines the ratio of cash to noncash (fringe benefits) compensation that an employer will pay to its employees?

2. What are the consequences if an employer raises its prices to pay for their employees' rising medical costs?

3. How is it possible for automobile employees in Michigan to receive more costly health benefits than automobile employees in the South, and yet automobiles produced in both locations sell for the same price?

4. Even if employees bear the entire cost (in terms of lower cash wages) of rising medical costs, why should employers still be concerned with cost containment?

5. Evaluate the following statement: "Rising medical costs are harmful to the economy because greater consumption expenditures on medical services results in lower savings, hence reduced private investment."

6. Evaluate the following statement: "Rising Medicare and Medicaid expenditures contribute to the growing federal deficit. To finance this larger deficit, the government must borrow more, which in turn increases interest rates, raises the value of the dollar, and consequently makes U.S. goods more expensive than foreign-produced goods."

Chapter 18. Why Is It So Difficult to Get into Medical School?

1. Evaluate the performance of the current market for medical education in terms of the number of qualified students admitted and the cost (both medical education and student forgone income) of becoming a physician.

2. The current approach for subsidizing medical schools results in all medical students being subsidized. Contrast this approach with one that awards the same amount of subsidy directly to students (according to their family incomes) for use in any medical school.

3. Medical schools are typically interested in "prestige." How would medical school behavior change if they had to survive in a competitive market (with free entry) and without subsidies?

4. An important reason why there are so few family practitioners is that their economic returns are so much lower than those of specialists. How would a competitive market in medical education increase the relative profitability of becoming a family practitioner?

5. Currently, the public is protected from incompetent and unethical physicians by requiring graduation from an approved medical school, passing a one-time licensing examination, and continuing education. What are alternative, lower-cost approaches for achieving these objectives?

Chapter 19. The Shortage of Nurses

1. Why has the demand for registered nurses been rising faster than its supply during the 1980s?

2. How have the last several shortages of nurses been resolved?

3. How does an increase in nurses' wages affect both hospitals' demand for nurses and the supply of nurses?

4. Why was the shortage of nurses that occurred before Medicare different from subsequent shortages?

5. Contrast the following two approaches for eliminating the shortage of nurses:

   a. Federal subsidies to nursing schools

   b. Increasing information on nurse demand and supply to prospective nursing students and to demanders of nursing services, such as hospitals

Chapter 20. The High Price of Prescription Drugs

1. Describe how the purchaser side of the drug prescription market is changing.

2. What are the advantages and disadvantages of quicker FDA approval of new drugs?

3. How valid an explanation for rising drug prices is the fact that research and development costs of new drugs have increased?

4. What are two possible explanations why the drug price index may not be an accurate indicator of drug price inflation.

5. Evaluate the assumptions underlying the following statement: "Differences in new drug prices reflect differences in their therapeutic benefits."

6. Would you prefer to see rising or constant new drug prices?

Chapter 21. Should Kidneys (and Other Organs) Be Bought and Sold?

1. Why have voluntary methods for increasing the supply of body organs been unsuccessful?

2. Evaluate the following proposal: Individuals would be permitted to sell the rights to their organs (in the form of reduced health or auto insurance premiums) if they were to die in an accident in the coming year.

3. Would government expenditures for kidney disease (currently covered as part of Medicare for all persons) be higher or lower under a free market system for kidneys?

4. Would the poor be disadvantaged to the benefit of those who are wealthy under a free market system for sale of kidneys?

5. Would it be more equitable if in a free market for sale of kidneys the poor were prohibited from selling their kidneys?

Chapter 22. The Role of Government in Medical Care

1. What were the dissatisfactions with the public interest view of government?

2. Contrast the benefit-cost calculations of legislators under both the public interest and economic theories of government.

3. Why are concentrated interests and diffuse costs important in predicting legislative outcomes?

4. Contrast the predictions of the public interest and economic theories of government with regard to redistributive policies.

5. Evaluate the following policies according to the two differing theories of government:
   a. Medicare and Medicaid: beneficiaries, taxation, and generosity of benefits
   b. The performance of state licensing boards in monitoring physician quality

Chapter 23. Medical Research, Medical Education, Alcohol Consumption, and Pollution: Who Should Pay?

1. What is the economist's definition of the correct or optimal rate of output?

2. Why do externalities, such as air and water pollution, occur?

3. Why do economists believe there is an optimal amount of pollution? What would occur if all pollution were eliminated?

4. Explain the rationale for requiring everyone who can afford it to purchase catastrophic health insurance.

5. The number of medical school spaces in this country is limited. Would there be fewer physicians if government subsidies for medical education were reduced?

Chapter 24. The Canadian Health Care System

1. Describe the Canadian health care system and the methods used to control costs.

2. What are the consequences of making medical services free to everyone?

3. Why is the size of administrative expenses (as a percent of total medical expenditures) a poor indication of a health care system's efficiency?

4. What are the "costs" (negative effects) of expenditure limits?

5. Contrast the criteria used in Canada and in competitive managed care systems for deciding whether an investment should be made in new technology.

Chapter 25. Employer-Mandated National Health Insurance

1. Why are employees in small firms less likely to have health insurance?

2. Would it be equitable to provide all employees in small firms with a subsidy for the purchase of health insurance?

3. What is likely to be the effect of employer-mandated health insurance on the employer's demand for labor?

4. Is an employer-mandated health insurance "tax" regressive, proportional, or progressive on the incomes of employees and consumers?

5. Which groups favor and which groups oppose an employer mandate for achieving national health insurance? Why?

Chapter 26. National Health Insurance: Which Approach and Why?

1. Discuss the criteria that should be used for evaluating alternative NHI proposals.

2. Evaluate the desirability of the following types of taxes for financing NHI: payroll, sales, and income taxes.

3. What is the justification for requiring everyone (all those who can afford it) to purchase a minimum level of health insurance?

4. Outline (and justify) a proposal for NHI. As part of your proposal, discuss the benefit package, beneficiaries, the method of financing, delivery of services, and the role of government. How well does your proposal meet the criteria discussed earlier?

5. What are alternative ways for treating Medicare under NHI?

Chapter 27. Financing Long-Term Care

1. What are the demographic and economic trends affecting the outlook for long-term care?

2. What should be the objectives of a long-term care policy? How do these objectives differ from the long-term care goals of the middle class?

3. Evaluate the redistributive effects of "front end" and "back end" government subsidies for nursing home care.

4. Evaluate the redistributive effects of income-related refundable tax credits for private long-term care insurance and medical individual retirement accounts.

5. Why has the market for long-term care insurance grown so slowly?

6. Why does private long-term care insurance, when sold to the aged, have such a high loading charge relative to the pure premium?

Chapter 28. The Politics of Health Care Reform

1. What are alternative hypotheses as to what NHI should achieve?

2. Why are groups that have a "concentrated interest" in particular legislation likely to be more influential in the policy process than groups that have a "diffuse interest" in the legislation's outcome?

3. How have medical and hospital associations influenced provider payment and delivery systems? Provide specific examples.

4. Discuss the goals of the major groups that have a concentrated interest in health care reform.

5. Why would an employer mandated NHI plan be insufficient, by itself, to secure the political support of the middle class?

6. Why is the structure and financing of any NHI plan likely to be inefficient and inequitable?

Index

Organ donors: compensation for, 220–25; "presumed consent" laws for, 220; signed cards for, 220; voluntary, 218–20
Organ transplants: centers for, 225; legislation of, 218, 220; Medicare coverage of, 217–18; number of, 217–18, *218, 219;* sources of organs for, 218–20. *See also* Organ donors
Outpatient care, 134, 198

Patients: as informed purchasers, 42–43; physicians as agents of, 35–36, 40–41; waiting times of, 156, 157, 249–50
Payroll taxes, 81–83, 264
Pepper Commission, 257
Physician incomes: in Canada, 248; changes in, 95–98, *96, 97, 98, 100;* future of, 102–5; private insurance and, 101; by specialty, *97;* technological innovations and, 101–2
Physicians: continuing education for, 190; demand for, 100–101; demand inducement by, 36–39, 42–43, 87, 91–92, 155; disciplinary actions for, 189; hospitals' interdependency with, 134–35; licensing of, 189–91; in managed care organizations, 40–41, 51–52, 103, 164–66; in medical groups, 103–5; monitoring of, 42–43, 112–15, 116–17, 187–88, 189–91, 247–48; motivations of, 35–43; national health insurance and, 294–95; peer review of, 188; as perfect agents of the patient, 35–36, 40–41; political power of, 292; price sensitivity faced by, 49–50; RBRVS and, 88–89, *90;* specialists, *90,* 91–92, 103–5, 190–

91; supply of, 8, 36–37, *37,* 39, 97. *See also* Malpractice; Medical schools; Physician incomes
Point-of-service (POS) plans, 162–64
Pollution: external costs of, 230, 244–45; health effects of, 26
POS. *See* Point-of-service plans
PPOs. *See* Preferred provider organizations
Preexisting conditions, 68–69
Preferred provider organizations (PPOs): definition of, 162, 163; demand inducement and, 40; growth of, 9, 102–3. *See also* Managed care organizations
Preferred-risk selection, 70–72, 84
Prescription drugs: comparisons of, by country, 211–12, *212;* direct patient payments for, *206;* FDA approval of, 213–14; formularies for, 208, 209–10; improvements in, 208–9; insurance for, 207; legislation of, 209–12; Medicaid and, 209–10; price controls on, 211–12; price index of, *205, 209,* 215–16; production costs of, 204, 206–7; research and development of, 204, 206–7, 211–12, 213–14; rising prices of, 204, 206–9; volume purchasers of, 207–8, 210
Price competition, 9, 123–29
Price controls: on medical expenditures, 151–59; on physicians under Medicare, 9; on prescription drugs, 211–12; in theory, 152–54. *See also* Resource-based relative value scale
Price discrimination, 146–48
Price sensitivity, 49–50, 146
Price setting, 140–41, *142,* 143–49

Rationing: by ability to pay, 45–46, 52–53; by government, 44–45,

About the Author

Paul J. Feldstein is a professor and FHP Foundation Distinguished Chair in Health Care Management at the Graduate School of Management, University of California, Irvine, since 1987. His previous position was at the University of Michigan as a professor in both the Department of Economics and the School of Public Health. Before that he was the director of the Division of Research at the American Hospital Association.

Professor Feldstein received his Ph.D. from the University of Chicago.

Professor Feldstein has written six books and over 60 articles on health care. His book *Health Care Economics*, 4th ed., is one of the most widely used texts on health economics. His book *The Politics of Health Legislation: An Economic Perspective* uses economic analysis to explain the outcome of health legislation in terms of the interest groups affected.

During several leaves from the university, Professor Feldstein worked at the Office of Management and Budget, the Social Security Administration, and the World Health Organization. He has been a consultant to many government and private health agencies, an expert witness on health antitrust issues, as well as serving on the board of Sutter Health, a large not-for-profit health care organization. Professor Feldstein's current research interests are on the reasons for the rapid increase in health insurance premiums and an examination of the effect of insurance company cost-containment programs, such as utilization review, on health insurance premiums and employee use of services. This research is being funded by the Robert Wood Johnson Foundation.

Other Books Published by
Health Administration Press
▼▼▼▼▼▼▼▼▼▼▼▼▼▼▼▼

HEALTH POLICYMAKING IN THE UNITED STATES
By Beaufort B. Longest, Jr.

This new book presents a basic model of the healthcare policymaking process that integrates the various and sometimes competing interests of our society. The author illustrates how policies are formulated, implemented, and modified.

The book covers the following topics: the definition of health policy and the way policies affect the health of our society, political dimensions of the policymaking process, the formulation of policy and the legislative process, how policies are implemented and changed, and the political interests of various parties in the policymaking process. The author also discusses how future healthcare policy is likely to be affected by the political marketplace and the U.S. economy.

Hardbound, 215 pages, August 1994, $38.00, Order No. 0947, ISBN 1-56793-017-4. An AUPHA/HAP Book

RURAL HEALTH SERVICES: A Management Perspective
Edited by Joyce E. Beaulieu and David E. Berry

With an emphasis on rural health services organization, this new book brings an up-to-date mix of research and practice into a well-drawn analysis of growing issues for the 90s and beyond as it examines America's underserved rural health delivery system.

The two-part narrative divides first into a comprehensive description and analysis of rural populations, the rural environment, and rural health policy organization and delivery during the early 1990s. The second part addresses issues of particular concern in planning, developing, administering, and evaluating rural health services. Emphasized are current practical policy and delivery issues concerning access to rural primary care services and services for the elderly and disabled.

Softbound, 298 pages, August 1994, $37.00, Order No. 0948, ISBN 1-56793-018-2. An AUPHA/HAP Book

CREATING NEW HOSPITAL–PHYSICIAN COLLABORATION
By Todd S. Wirth and Seth Allcorn

This book addresses a key strategy for hospital survival in the 1990s–the formation of partnerships between hospitals and physician medical groups. The authors examine integrated relationships and describe in detail methods for effectively managing these new networks. This book begins with a discussion of the economics of medical practice, the healthcare market, and the controls on healthcare delivery, showing motivations for healthcare executives and physicians to work together more closely. The second section concentrates on the management and business operations of medical groups and explores physician behavior, legal and political concerns, and the functioning of group practices. The last section offers specific approaches to hospital–physician affiliations.

Hardbound, 185 pages, 1993, $37.00, Order No. 0931, ISBN 0-910701-96-2. An American College of Healthcare Executives Management Series Book

INFORMATION SYSTEMS FOR HEALTH SERVICES ADMINISTRATION, 4th Edition
By Charles J. Austin, contributions by Charles J. Austin, Jr.

Indispensable for understanding and effectively using computerized hospital and health services information systems. This guide provides a thorough analysis of these management planning and control tools, examining hardware and software concepts, design and analysis, and technical applications. Two new chapters–"Information Systems Planning" and "Systems to Support Strategic Management and Planning"–have been added. The four part organization is as follows: Introduction and Background Concepts; Computing Technology; Systems Analysis, Design, Acquisition, and Implementation; and Health Services Applications of Computers. Discussion questions and additional readings accompany each chapter.

Hardbound, 341 pages, 1992, $41.00, Order No. 0917, ISBN 0-910701-83-0. An AUPHA/HAP Book

EVALUATING THE MEDICAL CARE SYSTEM:
Effectiveness, Efficiency, and Equity

By Lu Ann Aday, Charles E. Begley, David R. Lairson, and Carl H. Slater, with a foreword by Stephen M. Shortell

An introductory text for faculty and students in public health and health administration programs, this book defines and integrates the fundamental concepts and methods of health services research and illustrates their application to policy analysis. The authors apply the concepts and methods of epidemiology, economics, sociology, and other disciplines to illustrate the measurement and relevance of the effectiveness, efficiency, and equity criteria in evaluating healthcare system performance. They also cite specific examples of the significance of health services research in addressing contemporary health policy problems. This book provides a useful framework for understanding outcomes research and offers a comprehensive scope of the three dimensions for assessing care at the system level.

Softbound, 222 pages, June 1993, $32.00, Order No. 0933, ISBN 0-910701-98-9. An AHSR/HAP Book

MANAGED CARE IN MEDICAID:
Lessons for Policy and Program Design
By Robert E. Hurley, Deborah A. Freund, and John E. Paul

This new book chronicles and explores a decade of Medicaid reform initiatives–specifically those relating to primary care case management (PCCM). The authors evaluate three sets of managed care programs likely to be adopted. These programs are compared and contrasted in terms of: important cost, access, and quality implications; potential effect on provider participation; controversial restrictions on beneficiary choice of provider; and substantial investment of funds by federal and state governments. This book provides its readers with a thorough examination of the PCCM option at a time when the U.S. healthcare system is in transition and interest in managed care is intensified.

Softbound, 215 pages, 1993, $35.00, Order No. 0930, ISBN 0-910701-95-4 An AHSR/HAP Book

A Health Administration Press Journal

▼▼ ▼▼▼▼▼▼▼▼▼▼▼▼▼▼▼ ▼

FRONTIERS OF HEALTH SERVICES MANAGEMENT

The ideal guide for busy executives, each quarterly issue is a collection of forecasts and perspectives on one of today's emerging healthcare topics. Past issues have discussed regional hospital systems, effective governance in the 1990s, universal health insurance, trends in hospital–physician relationships, future health personnel issues, strategic alliance management, and total quality management.

Subscriptions: $65.00/year in the U.S.; $75.00 in Canada and all other countries. ISSN 0748-8157.

BOOK ORDERING INFORMATION

All Health Administration Press Publications are sent on a 30-day approval. To order call, (312) 943-0544, ext. 3000 or send your order to The Foundation of the American College of Healthcare Executives, Order Processing Center, Dept FE94, 1951 Cornell Avenue, Melrose Park, IL 60160-1001.

JOURNAL SUBSCRIPTION INFORMATION

Health Administration Press offers a money-back guarantee on all journal subscriptions. If you are not completely satisfied, simply write and cancel your subscription, you will receive a refund on all unmailed issues. Multi-year subscriptions are not available.

Please send checks made payable to the name of the publication for subscriptions. Current rates expire on December 31, 1995. Address orders to: The Foundation of the American College of Healthcare Executives, Order Processing Center, Dept. FE94, 1951 Cornell Avenue, Melrose Park, IL 60160-1001. Or for more information, call: (312) 943-0544, ext. 3000.

▼▼▼▼▼▼▼▼▼▼▼▼▼▼▼▼▼▼

2981 032